PREDIABETES DIET AND ACTION PLAN

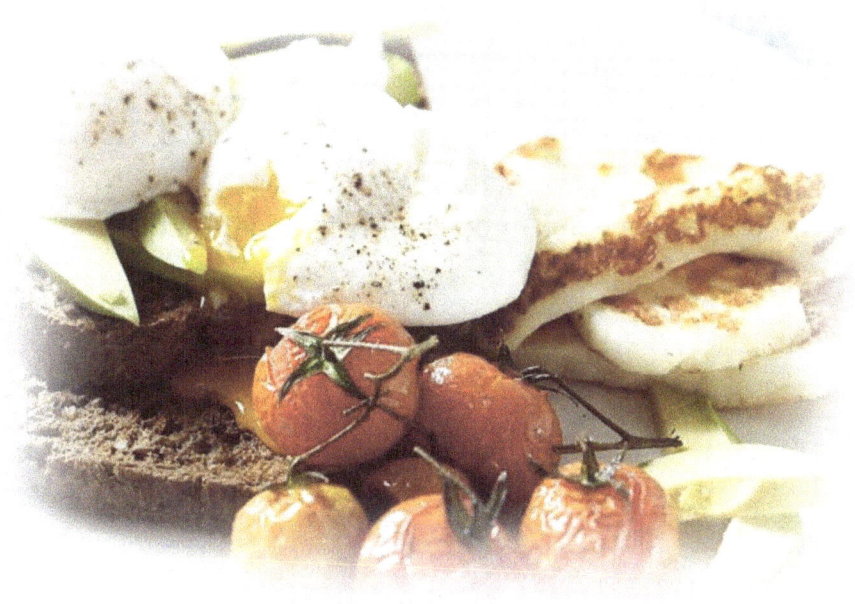

A Guide to Reversing Diabetes with Easy, Delicious Recipes.

Dr. Steven A.

Copyright © 2024 Dr. Steven A.

All rights reserved. No part of this book may be reproduced, stored in a retrieval system, or transmitted in any form or by any means, electronic, mechanical, photocopying, recording, scanning, or otherwise, without the publisher's prior written permission.

TABLE OF CONTENTS

PART I: FOUNDATIONS OF PREDIABETES REVERSAL 4

INTRODUCTION 5

CHAPTER 1: UNDERSTANDING PREDIABETES 7

- DEFINING PREDIABETES AND ITS IMPLICATIONS 7
- STATISTICS AND TRENDS IN PREDIABETES DIAGNOSIS 9
- RISK FACTORS AND COMMON MISCONCEPTIONS 10

CHAPTER 2: NUTRITION STRATEGIES FOR PREDIABETES MANAGEMENT 13

- THE ROLE OF CARBOHYDRATES, PROTEINS, AND FATS 13
- INTEGRATING CARBOHYDRATES, PROTEINS, AND FATS 16
- GLYCEMIC INDEX AND ITS IMPACT ON BLOOD SUGAR 17
- MEAL TIMING AND PORTION CONTROL 21

CHAPTER 3: PHYSICAL ACTIVITY AND PREDIABETES 25

- BENEFITS OF EXERCISE FOR PREDIABETES REVERSAL 25
- TYPES OF EXERCISE AND THEIR EFFECTS ON BLOOD SUGAR 26
- INCORPORATING PHYSICAL ACTIVITY INTO DAILY LIFE 26
- THREE WEEKS EXERCISE PLANS FOR PREDIABETES WITH HEALTH BENEFITS AND SAMPLE TEXT ILLUSTRATION 27

CHAPTER 4: MENTAL HEALTH, SLEEP, AND PREDIABETES 31

- STRESS MANAGEMENT TECHNIQUES AND THEIR ROLE IN BLOOD SUGAR CONTROL 31
- IMPORTANCE OF QUALITY SLEEP FOR METABOLIC HEALTH 32
- EFFECTS OF SLEEP DEPRIVATION ON METABOLIC HEALTH: 34
- MINDFULNESS PRACTICES AND THEIR IMPACT ON PREDIABETES 34

PART II: MEAL PLAN AND RECIPES 36

CHAPTER 5: CREATING A 3-WEEK PREDIABETES REVERSAL PLAN — 37

- DESIGNING BALANCED MEALS AND SNACKS — 37
- SAMPLE MEAL PLANS FOR BREAKFAST, LUNCH, DINNER, AND SNACKS — 40
- GROCERY SHOPPING TIPS AND INGREDIENT SUBSTITUTIONS — 43

BREAKFASTS AND SMOOTHIES — 45

- NUTRIENT-DENSE BREAKFAST OPTIONS FOR BLOOD SUGAR CONTROL — 46
- ENERGIZING SMOOTHIE RECIPES FOR PREDIABETES MANAGEMENT — 49
- MEAL PREP TIPS FOR BUSY MORNINGS — 52
- AVOIDED BREAKFASTS AND SMOOTHIES: — 52

SALADS AND LIGHT MAINS — 53

- WHOLESOME SALAD RECIPES PACKED WITH FIBER AND FLAVOR — 54
- QUICK AND EASY MEAL SOLUTIONS FOR BUSY WEEKNIGHTS — 60
- AVOIDED SALADS AND LIGHT MAINS — 62

HEARTY MAINS — 63

- PROTEIN-RICH DINNER RECIPES FOR PREDIABETES REVERSAL — 64
- VEGETARIAN AND PLANT-BASED OPTIONS FOR HEART HEALTH — 67
- COOKING TECHNIQUES TO ENHANCE FLAVOR WITHOUT SACRIFICING NUTRITION — 70
- AVOIDED HEARTY MAINS — 70

SNACKS, SIDES, AND SWEETS — 71

- WHOLESOME SNACK IDEAS TO KEEP BLOOD SUGAR STABLE BETWEEN MEALS — 72
- AVOIDED SNACKS — 74
- FLAVORFUL SIDE DISH RECIPES TO COMPLEMENT ANY MEAL — 75
- AVOIDED SIDES — 77
- INDULGENT DESSERT OPTIONS FOR OCCASIONAL TREATS — 78
- AVOIDED SWEETS — 80

CONCLUSION — 81

PART I: FOUNDATIONS OF PREDIABETES REVERSAL

INTRODUCTION

Imagine living a life where you are constantly on the edge of developing a chronic condition that threatens your health, energy, and overall well-being. Prediabetes is that silent alarm warning you that your body is teetering on the brink of a more serious health crisis. The good news? It's not too late to turn things around. With the proper knowledge and actionable plan, you can reclaim control over your health and steer clear of diabetes.

Prediabetes Diet and Action Plan: A Guide to Reversing Diabetes with Easy, Delicious Recipes is designed to be your comprehensive guide on this journey. This book covers the vital aspects of managing and reversing prediabetes, focusing on nutrition, physical activity, mental health, and lifestyle changes. The themes revolve around practical strategies, scientific insights, and real-world applications that empower you to take charge of your health.

Prediabetes affects millions of people worldwide, often without them even knowing. It's a condition that signals a higher risk of developing type 2 diabetes, heart disease, and stroke. By addressing prediabetes early, you can prevent these severe health issues. This book is crucial because it provides theoretical knowledge and actionable steps to implement immediately to improve your health outcomes. Understanding and managing prediabetes can be life-changing, and this book aims to make that transformation accessible to everyone.

As an expert dietitian, I have seen firsthand how lifestyle changes can dramatically alter the course of prediabetes. My perspective is rooted in professional experience and a bottomless commitment to helping individuals achieve their best health. This book is a distillation of research, patient interactions, and successful outcomes, all aimed at providing the tools you need to succeed.

This book posits that with the proper diet, exercise regimen, and lifestyle adjustments, prediabetes can not only be managed but reversed. Following the comprehensive action plan outlined in these pages can reduce your risk of developing diabetes and improve your overall health.

The structure of the book is designed to guide you step-by-step through your journey of reversing prediabetes:

Foundations of Prediabetes Reversal:
- Understanding prediabetes and its implications
- Nutrition strategies for blood sugar management
- The importance of physical activity
- The role of mental health and sleep

Meal Plan and Recipes:
- A practical two-week meal plan
- Nutritious and delicious breakfast and smoothie recipes
- Wholesome salads and light mains
- Hearty main courses for dinner
- Healthy snacks, sides, and sweets

Each chapter has practical tips, scientific explanations, and real-life examples to help you integrate these changes seamlessly into your life.

As you turn each page, you will find a treasure trove of information that will change how you view food, exercise, and self-care. Discover why certain foods impact your blood sugar levels more than others, learn effective stress management techniques that stabilize your glucose levels, and explore the power of quality sleep in maintaining metabolic health.

You might wonder, "Is this another diet book that makes promises it can't keep?" This is not a fad diet book filled with unrealistic expectations. Every strategy, tip, and recipe in this book is backed by scientific research and proven results. The goal is not just short-term fixes but long-lasting changes that become a natural part of your daily life.

CHAPTER 1: UNDERSTANDING PREDIABETES

Defining Prediabetes and Its Implications

Prediabetes. It's a term that's been gaining traction in recent years, cropping up in conversations with healthcare providers and popping up in health-related articles and news segments. But what exactly is prediabetes, and why should it matter to you? Let's unpack this concept together, peeling back the layers to reveal its significance and implications for your health and well-being.

At its core, prediabetes is a condition characterized by higher-than-normal blood sugar levels, yet not relatively high enough to be diagnosed as type 2 diabetes. It's often described as a "warning sign" or a "wake-up call" from your body, signaling that you're at increased risk of developing full-blown diabetes if left unchecked. Picture it as a yellow caution light flashing on your dashboard, urging you to slow down and take notice before you reach the red zone.

But what do these high blood sugar levels mean for your health? They're a red flag indicating that your body struggles to regulate glucose properly, the primary energy source for your cells. When you eat, carbohydrates from your food are broken down into glucose, then transported through your bloodstream to fuel your cells. However, in prediabetes, this process becomes somewhat derailed. Your cells become resistant to the effects of insulin, a hormone produced by your pancreas that helps usher glucose into your cells. As a result, glucose levels in your bloodstream remain high for more extended periods, leading to a condition known as hyperglycemia.

You might wonder, "So what if my blood sugar levels are slightly high? What's the big deal?" Ah, but here's where the plot thickens. High blood sugar levels, even if they haven't crossed the threshold into diabetes territory, can wreak havoc on your body over time. Think of it as a slow and stealthy intruder, gradually undermining your health from within.

First and foremost, prediabetes is a significant risk factor for the development of type 2 diabetes, the more familiar cousin of prediabetes. Studies have shown that up to 70% of individuals with prediabetes will eventually progress to type 2 diabetes if they don't take proactive steps to intervene. This transition isn't just a minor inconvenience – it's a life-altering diagnosis that comes with a laundry list of potential complications, including heart disease, stroke, kidney damage, nerve damage, and vision loss.

But wait, there's more. Prediabetes isn't enough to stop diabetes. Oh no, it's also cozying up to other unsavory characters in the chronic disease lineup, including obesity, hypertension, and dyslipidemia (abnormal cholesterol levels and fats in the blood). It's like a domino effect, with one health issue knocking into the next, setting off a cascade of consequences that can significantly impact your quality of life.

And here's the kicker – prediabetes often flies under the radar, masquerading as a benign condition until it's too late. Many people with prediabetes don't experience any symptoms, or they may attribute their symptoms to other factors, like stress or aging. This stealth mode of operation makes prediabetes a particularly insidious foe, waiting in the shadows until it decides to make its grand entrance onto the main stage of your health.

But fear not, dear reader, for all is not lost. While prediabetes may sound like a dire diagnosis, it also presents a golden opportunity for intervention and prevention. By taking proactive steps to address prediabetes early on, you can significantly reduce your risk of developing type 2 diabetes and its associated complications. It's like hitting the pause button on the progression of the disease, giving yourself a fighting chance to rewrite the script of your health story.

So, what does it all boil down to? Prediabetes is more than just a buzzword—it's a critical turning point in your health journey, signaling the need for action and empowerment. It's a wake-up call to tune in to the signals your body is sending and heed the warnings before they escalate into something more serious. Above all, it's a reminder that you can shape your destiny, reclaim control of your health, and rewrite your life's narrative.

Statistics and Trends in Prediabetes Diagnosis

A landscape spread with data points, each a snapshot of a growing health crisis that threatens millions worldwide. It's a tale of numbers, but behind each statistic lies a human story, a life touched by the shadow of prediabetes.

To truly grasp the magnitude of our predicament, we must first understand the scale of the problem. Prediabetes isn't just a niche issue affecting a handful of individuals – it's a widespread phenomenon that's reaching epidemic proportions. According to the Centers for Disease Control and Prevention (C.D.C.), an estimated 97.6 million American adults – that's more than one in three – have prediabetes.

But wait, it gets even more alarming. Despite the staggering prevalence of prediabetes, awareness of the condition remains shockingly low. A study published in the Journal of the American Medical Association found that nearly 90% of individuals with prediabetes were unaware of their condition. That's right – the vast majority of people walking around with high blood sugar levels have no idea that they're at increased risk of developing type 2 diabetes.

So, why is prediabetes flying under the radar? Part of the problem lies in the subtle nature of the condition. Unlike diabetes, which often presents with noticeable symptoms like excessive thirst, frequent urination, and unexplained weight loss, prediabetes is frequently asymptomatic. People may feel perfectly fine and assume everything is hunky-dory with their health, unaware of the silent storm beneath the surface.

Another contributing factor is the lack of routine screening for prediabetes in primary care settings. Unlike other routine tests like cholesterol screenings or blood pressure checks, there's no standardised protocol for screening for prediabetes during routine medical exams. As a result, many individuals with prediabetes slip through the cracks, their condition going undetected until it's too late.

But it's not just a lack of awareness and screening that's fueling the prediabetes epidemic. It's also a perfect storm of societal factors that are contributing to the rise in prediabetes rates. Our modern way of life, characterised by sedentary behavior, poor dietary choices, and chronic stress, has created the ideal breeding ground for metabolic dysfunction. Fast food joints on every corner, seductive screens beckoning us to sit and scroll for hours on end, and the relentless pace of modern life is a recipe for disaster in our health.

And let's remember the role of genetics in the prediabetes puzzle. While lifestyle factors certainly play a significant role in the development of prediabetes, genetics also exert a powerful influence on our susceptibility to the condition. Some individuals may have a genetic predisposition to insulin resistance, making them more prone to developing prediabetes even in the absence of overt lifestyle risk factors.

So, where do we go from here? How do we stem the tide of prediabetes and prevent it from morphing into full-blown diabetes? The answer lies in awareness, education, and proactive intervention. We must spotlight prediabetes, bringing it out of the shadows and into the forefront of public consciousness. We must empower individuals to take charge of their health, arming them with the knowledge and resources they need to make informed decisions about their lifestyle habits. We must also invest in initiatives to promote healthy behaviors and create environments that support health and well-being.

Risk Factors and Common Misconceptions

First, let's tackle the elephant in the room – what exactly are the risk factors for prediabetes? Contrary to popular belief, prediabetes isn't a one-size-fits-all condition. It doesn't discriminate based on age, gender, or socioeconomic status. Instead, a multifaceted interplay of genetic, environmental, and lifestyle factors converges to elevate your risk of developing high blood sugar levels.

One of the most well-established risk factors for prediabetes is excess weight, particularly around the abdomen. Belly fat isn't just a harmless cushioning – it's a metabolically active tissue that churns out hormones and inflammatory substances, disrupting your body's delicate balance of insulin and glucose. As your waistline expands, so too does your risk of prediabetes.

But weight isn't the only player in the prediabetes game. Genetics also play a significant role in determining your susceptibility to the condition. If you have a family history of diabetes, particularly in a parent or sibling, your risk of developing prediabetes is significantly high. It's like inheriting a genetic time bomb, ticking away silently in the background, waiting for the right moment to detonate.

Also, remember the age. As we grow older, our risk of developing prediabetes naturally increases. This isn't just a consequence of aging. It also reflects the cumulative impact of years of lifestyle habits, dietary choices, and metabolic changes accumulated over time. It's like a slow and steady march toward metabolic dysfunction, with each passing year bringing us closer to the brink of prediabetes.

But here's where things get interesting – not all risk factors for prediabetes are set in stone. Some are within our control, while others are beyond our influence. Take, for example, lifestyle factors like diet and physical activity. A diet high in refined carbohydrates, saturated fats, and sugary beverages can significantly increase your risk of prediabetes, while regular exercise can help mitigate that risk. It's like a game of balancing scales, with each choice tipping the odds in favour of health or disease.

Yet despite the abundance of scientific evidence supporting the role of lifestyle in prediabetes risk, there are still common misconceptions that persist. One of the most pervasive myths is that prediabetes is a benign condition that doesn't warrant serious attention. Nothing could be further from the truth. Prediabetes is a serious warning sign for your body, signaling that your metabolic machinery is out of whack and in need of recalibration. Ignoring it won't make it disappear – it will only allow it to progress unchecked, laying the groundwork for more serious health complications.

Another common misconception is that prediabetes is solely a result of poor dietary choices and lack of exercise. While lifestyle factors are significant, they're only part of the equation. Genetics, age, and other underlying health conditions can also influence your risk of developing prediabetes, making it a complex and multifactorial condition that defies simple explanations.

So, what's the takeaway from all of this? Prediabetes isn't just a roll of the genetic dice or a consequence of poor lifestyle choices – it's a complex interplay of factors that converge to elevate your risk of developing high blood sugar levels. By understanding the risk factors and dispelling common misconceptions, we can empower ourselves to take proactive steps to prevent prediabetes and protect our long-term health. It's like shining a light into the darkness, illuminating the path to wellness and vitality for ourselves and future generations.

Thank you for purchasing "Prediabetes Diet and Action Plan: A Guide to Reversing Diabetes with Easy, Delicious Recipes." *Your decision to invest in your health and take proactive steps toward managing and reversing prediabetes is commendable.*

We hope this book's insights, strategies, and practical advice will empower you to better health. As an independent publisher, your feedback is invaluable to me. Your experiences, thoughts, and suggestions help improve the quality of my future work and assist other readers navigating similar health challenges.

Please take a moment to share your feedback. Your reviews and comments can make a significant difference in spreading awareness and helping others make informed decisions about managing prediabetes. Whether it's a personal story of success, a suggestion for improvement, or your thoughts on the book, your input is deeply appreciated.

Thank you again for your support, and I wish you the best on your journey to optimal health.

Warm regards,

[Dr. Steven A.]

CHAPTER 2: NUTRITION STRATEGIES FOR PREDIABETES MANAGEMENT

The Role of Carbohydrates Proteins and Fats

Crossing the world of nutrition can be discouraging, especially when you're faced with a diagnosis of prediabetes. This condition, a precursor to type 2 diabetes, signals that your blood sugar levels are higher than average but not yet high enough to be classified as diabetes. The good news? With the right dietary strategies, you can manage and even reverse prediabetes.

Carbohydrates: The Double Edged

Primary Energy Source:

- Carbohydrates are the body's preferred energy source, essential for fueling physical and cognitive functions. When consumed, they're broken down into glucose, which enters the bloodstream and is used by cells for energy.

- For those with prediabetes, it's crucial to manage carbohydrate intake to prevent spikes in blood sugar levels.

Glycemic Index and Load:

- Not all carbs are created equal. The glycemic index (G.I.) Indicate how quickly a carbohydrate-containing food increases blood sugar levels. Low-GI foods cause slower, more stable increases in blood sugar.

- Glycemic load (G.L.) considers both the G.I. and the portion size. Choosing foods with a low G.L. can help maintain stable blood sugar levels.

Types of Carbohydrates:

- **Simple Carbohydrates** Are found in sugary snacks, sodas, and processed foods. These are rapidly digested and can cause quick spikes in blood sugar.

- **Complex Carbohydrates** Are found in whole grains, vegetables, fruits, and legumes. These are digested more slowly, leading to a gradual release of glucose into the bloodstream.

Fiber:

- One kind of carbohydrate that the body is unable to process is fiber. It helps regulate blood sugar levels by slowing down the absorption of sugar, and it also promotes satiety and digestive health.

- Whole grains, fruits, vegetables, and legumes are foods high in fiber.

Proteins: The Building Blocks of Health

Muscle Repair and Growth:

- Proteins are necessary for the repair and growth of tissues. They are critical in maintaining muscle mass and are essential for overall metabolism and glucose regulation.

- Consuming adequate protein helps prevent muscle loss, which can occur with age or weight loss efforts.

Satiety and Blood Sugar Control:

- Protein-rich foods can help control hunger and promote feelings of fullness, reducing the likelihood of overeating.

- Protein also has a minimal impact on blood sugar levels, making it a stable energy source.

Amino Acids:

- Proteins are composed of essential amino acids, some of which must be obtained through the diet.

- Animal sources like meat, poultry, fish, eggs, and dairy provide complete proteins containing all essential amino acids.
- Plant sources like beans, lentils, nuts, seeds, and grains can be combined to provide complete proteins.

Fats: The Essential Nutrient

Energy Storage and Insulation:

- Fats are a concentrated energy source, providing more than twice the calories per gram compared to carbohydrates and proteins.
- They shield the body's essential organs and provide insulation.

Essential Fatty Acids:

- Some fats are essential for health and must be obtained through the diet, such as omega-3 and omega-6 fatty acids.
- These fats are crucial for brain function, reducing inflammation, and supporting heart health.

Types of Fats:

- **Saturated Fats:** These are found in animal products and tropical oils. They should be limited as they can increase the risk of heart disease.
- **Trans Fats:** Found in many processed foods. These are harmful and should be avoided as much as possible.
- **Unsaturated Fats:** These are found in avocados, nuts, seeds, and fish. They are beneficial and can help improve blood cholesterol levels and reduce inflammation.

Role in Blood Sugar Control:

- Healthy fats can help slow the digestion of carbohydrates, leading to more stable blood sugar levels.
- Including a balance of fats in meals can help with satiety and prevent overeating.

Integrating Carbohydrates Proteins and Fats

Balancing carbohydrates, proteins, and fats in your diet is critical to managing prediabetes effectively. Here are some strategies to help you achieve this balance:

Balanced Meals:

- Aim to include all three macronutrients in every meal. This approach ensures a steady release of energy and prevents blood sugar spikes.
- For example, pair whole grains (carbohydrates) with lean protein (chicken, fish, tofu) and healthy fats (avocado, olive oil) to create a balanced plate.

Mindful Portions:

- Be mindful of serving sizes, particularly when it comes to carbohydrates. Blood sugar levels can be better managed with smaller meals.
- Use your plate as a guide: Fill half with non-starchy vegetables, one-quarter with protein, and one-quarter with whole grains or starchy vegetables.

Healthy Snacking:

- Choose snacks that combine protein, healthy fats, and fiber-rich carbohydrates. This combination helps keep you full between meals and maintains stable blood sugar levels.
- Examples include apple slices with peanut butter, Greek yoghurt with berries, or a handful of nuts with a piece of fruit.

Limit Processed Foods:

- Minimize the intake of processed and refined foods, often high in simple sugars and unhealthy fats.
- Focus on whole, nutrient-dense foods that provide sustained energy and essential nutrients.

Glycemic Index and Its Impact on Blood Sugar

The glycemic index is a powerful tool that can help you direct this world more effectively, turning your diet into a powerful ally in your fight for health. By understanding and utilising the glycemic index, you can take control of your blood sugar levels, making informed decisions that promote well-being and prevent the progression of diabetes.

Glycemic Index (G.I.):

Definition and Purpose:

- The glycemic index is a numerical system that measures how quickly carbohydrates in foods increase blood sugar levels. It ranks foods on a scale from 0 to 100 based on their immediate impact on blood glucose.

- Foods with a high G.I. cause rapid spikes in blood sugar, while those with a low G.I. result in a slower, more gradual increase. This information is critical for individuals managing prediabetes as it helps them choose foods that stabilize blood sugar levels.

High G.I. Foods:

- High G.I. foods have a score of 70 or above. These foods are rapidly digested and absorbed, causing a swift rise in blood sugar.

- Examples include white bread, sugary cereals, baked goods, and processed snacks.

- Consuming high G.I. foods frequently can lead to sharp blood sugar fluctuations, which strain the body's insulin response and increase the risk of developing type 2 diabetes.

Low G.I. Foods:

- Low G.I. foods have a score of 55 or below. These foods are digested and absorbed more slowly, leading to a gradual increase in blood sugar.
- Examples include whole grains, legumes, fruits and vegetables, and nuts.
- Incorporating low-G.I. foods into the diet helps maintain stable blood sugar levels, reduces the risk of insulin resistance, and aids in weight management.

Moderate G.I. Foods:

- Moderate G.I. foods fall between 56 and 69 on the glycemic index scale. These foods have a moderate impact on blood sugar levels.
- Examples include whole wheat products, brown rice, and certain fruits like bananas and grapes.
- While moderate G.I. foods can be included in a balanced diet, they should be consumed in moderation and paired with low G.I. foods to help maintain stable blood sugar levels.

Factors Influencing G.I.:

- Several factors influence the glycemic index of a food, including its carbohydrate type, fiber content, fat and protein composition, and cooking method.
- For instance, whole grains have a lower G.I. than refined grains because they contain more fiber, which slows digestion.
- Combining high G.I. foods with proteins or fats can lower their overall glycemic impact, as these macronutrients slow down the absorption of carbohydrates.

Impact on Blood Sugar:

Blood Sugar Control:

- Managing blood sugar is crucial for individuals with prediabetes, as fluctuating levels can lead to insulin resistance and increased risk of diabetes.

- By choosing low and moderate G.I. foods, you can prevent sharp spikes in blood sugar, promote more consistent energy levels, and reduce the burden on your pancreas to produce insulin.

Reducing Insulin Resistance:

- High blood sugar levels over time can lead to insulin resistance, where the body's cells become less responsive to insulin.

- A diet focused on low G.I. foods helps mitigate this risk by stabilising blood sugar levels, allowing the body's insulin to work more effectively.

Satiety and Weight Management:

- Low G.I. foods contribute to fullness and satisfaction, helping control appetite and reduce overall calorie intake.

- By stabilising blood sugar and reducing hunger pangs, these foods support weight management efforts, which are crucial for managing prediabetes and preventing type 2 diabetes.

Heart Health:

- High blood sugar levels and insulin resistance are linked to an increased risk of cardiovascular disease.

- Low G.I. foods help control blood sugar and support heart health by improving lipid profiles and reducing inflammation.

Emotional Well-being:

- Blood sugar fluctuations can significantly impact mood and energy levels, leading to irritability, fatigue, and even depression.
- By maintaining stable blood sugar through a low G.I. diet, individuals can experience more balanced moods and sustained energy, improving overall quality of life.

Practical Tips for Implementing G.I.:

Plan Balanced Meals:

- Create meals combining low-GI carbohydrates, proteins, and healthy fats to balance blood sugar levels. For example, pair whole-grain bread with avocado and eggs for a nutritious breakfast.
- Incorporate a variety of low-GI fruits and vegetables into your meals to increase fiber intake and enhance nutrient diversity.

Be Mindful of Portion Sizes:

- Even low G.I. foods can impact blood sugar if consumed in large quantities. Practice portion control to ensure balanced blood sugar levels throughout the day.
- Use smaller plates and focus on hunger and fullness cues to avoid overeating.

Choose Whole Foods Over Processed Foods:

- Opt for minimally processed foods like whole grains, legumes, and fresh produce, which typically have lower G.I. scores than their processed counterparts.
- Avoid sugary snacks, refined grains, and processed foods that can lead to blood sugar spikes and increased insulin demand.

Experiment with Cooking Methods:

- The way you prepare food can impact its glycemic index. For instance, al dente pasta has a lower G.I. than fully cooked pasta.

- Experiment with different cooking methods, such as steaming or grilling, to help maintain the integrity of the food's natural fibers and lower its G.I.

Incorporate Regular Physical Activity:

- Physical activity helps regulate blood sugar levels and enhances insulin sensitivity. Aim for at least 150 minutes of moderate weekly exercise, such as brisk walking, cycling, or swimming.

- Combine cardiovascular exercise with strength training to maximize blood sugar control and overall health benefits.

Meal Timing and Portion Control

Managing prediabetes can be an enlightening and challenging process. Two essential tactics become clear as we work to restore control over our health and stabilize blood sugar levels: meal scheduling and portion control. These methods support us in developing better eating habits and a more positive relationship with food while managing prediabetes.

Meal Timing:

- **Consistent Eating Schedule:** Regular eating helps stabilize blood sugar levels. Skipping meals can lead to overeating later and cause blood sugar spikes. Aim to eat roughly the exact times daily to keep your metabolism steady and your energy levels balanced.

- **Balanced Breakfast:** Starting the day with a balanced breakfast sets a positive tone for the rest of the day. Incorporate a mix of protein, healthy fats, and complex carbohydrates to provide sustained energy and prevent mid-morning blood sugar crashes. Consider Greek yoghurt with nuts and berries or a vegetable omelet with whole-grain toast.

- **Frequent, Smaller Meals:** Eating smaller, more frequent meals can prevent the significant blood sugar fluctuations that occur with larger, less frequent meals. Strive for three main meals and two to three small snacks throughout the day. This approach helps maintain steady glucose levels and reduces the risk of overeating.

- **Nighttime Eating:** Avoid late-night eating, as it can interfere with your body's ability to manage blood sugar levels overnight. Aim to finish your last meal at least two to three hours before bedtime. This practice supports better sleep quality and allows your body to rest and repair without the burden of digestion.

- **Post-Meal Activity:** Doing light physical activity after meals, such as a short walk, can help lower blood sugar levels. This simple habit enhances insulin sensitivity and aids in glucose regulation, providing a natural boost to your efforts in managing prediabetes.

Portion Control:

- **Mindful Eating:** Practice mindful eating by paying attention to your meals, savoring each bite, and recognising when you're full. This approach helps prevent overeating and allows you to enjoy your food more thoroughly. Turn off distractions like TV and focus on the sensory experience of eating.

- **Portion Awareness:** Use smaller plates and bowls to help control portion sizes. Visual cues, like a full smaller plate, can trick your brain into feeling satisfied with less food. Familiarizes yourself with standard portion sizes for different food groups to better gauge appropriate servings.

- **Balanced Plates:** A balanced plate should include a variety of food groups. Arrange your plate such that non-starchy veggies make up half of it, lean protein makes up the other quarter, and whole grains or starchy vegetables make up the last quarter. This visual aid makes sure you're eating a balanced, nutrient-rich meal.

- **Portion Size Tricks:** Implement portion control tricks like dividing restaurant meals in half and saving the rest for later or sharing large dishes with a friend. At home, pre-portion snacks into smaller containers rather than eating directly from the package to avoid mindless munching.

- **Hydration:** Sometimes, thirst can be mistaken for hunger. Stay well-hydrated by drinking plenty of water throughout the day. Before reaching for a snack, try drinking a glass of water and waiting a few minutes to see if your hunger subsides.

- **Protein and Fiber:** Incorporate more protein and fiber into your meals to promote satiety and reduce overall calorie intake. Protein and fiber-rich foods like beans, legumes, lean meats, and whole grains keep you fuller for longer and help manage blood sugar levels.
- **Slow Down:** Eat slowly and give your body time to register fullness. It takes about 20 minutes for your brain to signal that you're full, so pace yourself and savor each bite. This practice can prevent overeating and enhance your overall dining experience.

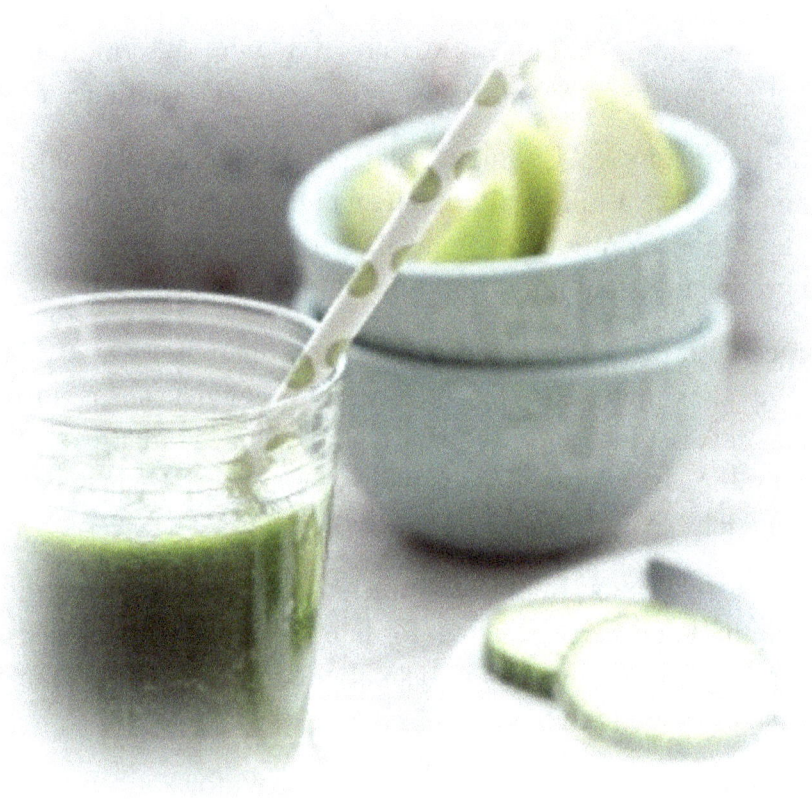

Thank You for Choosing "Prediabetes Diet and Action Plan"

Thank you for purchasing "Prediabetes Diet and Action Plan: A Guide to Reversing Diabetes with Easy, Delicious Recipes." Your decision to invest in your health and take proactive steps toward managing and reversing prediabetes is commendable.

We hope this book's insights, strategies, and practical advice will empower you to better health. As an independent publisher, your feedback is invaluable to me. Your experiences, thoughts, and suggestions help improve the quality of my future work and assist other readers navigating similar health challenges.

Please take a moment to share your feedback. Your reviews and comments can make a significant difference in spreading awareness and helping others make informed decisions about managing prediabetes. Whether it's a personal story of success, a suggestion for improvement, or your thoughts on the book, your input is deeply appreciated.

Thank you once again for your support. I wish you the best on your journey to optimal health.

Warm regards,

[Dr. Steven A]

CHAPTER 3: PHYSICAL ACTIVITY AND PREDIABETES

Physical activity plays a crucial role in the management and reversal of prediabetes. It involves any movement that expends energy, from structured exercise routines to everyday activities like walking or gardening. For individuals with prediabetes, regular physical activity can significantly improve blood sugar control, enhance insulin sensitivity, and support weight management.

Benefits of Exercise for Prediabetes Reversal

Regular exercise offers numerous benefits for individuals with prediabetes, including:

- **Improved Insulin Sensitivity:** Physical activity helps your body use insulin more effectively, allowing glucose to enter your cells and be used for energy, thus reducing blood sugar levels.

- **Weight Management:** Exercise aids in weight loss and weight maintenance, which can help improve insulin sensitivity and reduce the risk of developing type 2 diabetes.

- **Lowered Blood Sugar Levels:** Regular physical activity can lower fasting blood sugar levels and improve overall glycemic control.

- **Reduced Risk of Heart Disease:** Exercise helps lower blood pressure, improve cholesterol levels, and reduce the risk of cardiovascular disease, which is often associated with prediabetes.

- **Increased Energy Levels:** Regular physical activity can boost energy levels, improve mood, and reduce stress, leading to an overall sense of well-being.

Types of Exercise and Their Effects on Blood Sugar

Different types of exercise can have varying effects on blood sugar levels. Here are some common types of exercise and their impact:

- **Aerobic Exercise:** Activities like brisk walking, jogging, swimming, and cycling can help lower blood sugar levels by increasing insulin sensitivity and promoting muscle glucose uptake.

- **Strength Training:** Resistance exercises, such as weightlifting and bodyweight, can improve muscle mass and insulin sensitivity, improving blood sugar control over time.

- **Flexibility and Balance Exercises:** Practices like yoga, tai chi, and Pilates can improve flexibility, balance, and overall mobility, reducing the risk of falls and injuries.

- **Interval Training:** High-intensity interval training (HIIT) involves alternating between short bursts of intense activity and rest or low-intensity exercise periods. HIIT can be particularly effective for improving insulin sensitivity and burning calories in a shorter amount of time.

Incorporating Physical Activity into Daily Life

Making physical activity a part of your daily routine is essential for long-term success in prediabetes management. Here are some tips for incorporating exercise into your daily life:

- **Set Realistic Goals:** Start small and gradually increase the duration and intensity of your workouts over time. Aim for at least 150 minutes of moderate-intensity aerobic activity, 75 minutes of vigorous-intensity activity per week, and two or more days of strength training exercises.

- **Find Activities You Enjoy:** Choose activities you enjoy and look forward to doing. Whether dancing, hiking, gardening, or playing sports, find something that makes you feel good and fits your lifestyle.

- **Make It Social:** You may hold yourself accountable and have more fun working out with friends, family, or coworkers. Join a fitness class, sports team, or walking group to stay motivated and connected.

- **Incorporate Movement Throughout the Day:** Look for opportunities to be active throughout the day, such as taking the stairs instead of the elevator, parking farther away from your destination, or performing housework like vacuuming or gardening.

- **Listen to Your Body:** Pay attention to how your body feels during and after exercise. If you experience pain or discomfort, adjust your activities accordingly and consult with a healthcare professional if needed.

Three weeks exercise plan for prediabetes with health benefits and sample text illustration

NOTE:

"Unlock the life-changing benefits of regular exercise to take charge of prediabetes and elevate your well-being. Physical activity not only boosts insulin sensitivity and aids in weight management but also revitalizes your energy and lifts your spirits. You set the stage for a healthier, more vibrant future by weaving fun and engaging activities into your daily life. Each step brings you closer to overcoming prediabetes and living a life full of health and vitality."

Week 1: Getting Started

Day 1: Brisk Walking

- **Exercise:** Start with a 20-minute walk around your neighborhood or local park.

- **Health Benefits:** Brisk walking improves cardiovascular health, boosts mood, and helps lower blood sugar levels.

- **Illustration:** Put on your favorite sneakers, step outside, and walk at a pace that allows you to carry on a conversation but leaves you slightly breathless.

Day 2: Bodyweight Strength Training

- **Exercise:** Perform bodyweight exercises such as squats, lunges, push-ups, and planks for 15 minutes.

- **Health Benefits:** Strength training builds muscle mass, improves metabolism, and enhances insulin sensitivity.

- **Illustration:** Find a comfortable space at home, use a sturdy chair for support if needed, and perform each exercise with proper form and control.

Day 3: Yoga or Stretching

- **Exercise:** Practice yoga or perform a 15-minute stretching routine to improve flexibility and reduce stress.

- **Health Benefits:** Yoga reduces stress, promotes relaxation, and increases flexibility and balance.

- **Illustration:** Roll out a yoga mat, follow along with a guided yoga video, or stretch on your own, focusing on deep breathing and gentle movements

Week 2: Building Momentum
Day 4: Cycling or Stationary Biking

- **Exercise:** Go for a 30-minute bike ride outdoors or use a stationary bike at home or the gym.

- **Health Benefits:** Cycling improves cardiovascular health, strengthens leg muscles, and burns calories.

- **Illustration**: If cycling outdoors, wear a helmet and follow bike safety rules. If using a stationary bike, adjust the resistance to challenge yourself.

Day 5: High-Intensity Interval Training (HIIT)

- **Exercise:** Perform a 20-minute HIIT workout consisting of alternating periods of high-intensity exercise (e.g., jumping jacks, burpees) and rest.

- **Health Benefits:** HIIT boosts metabolism, burns fat, and improves cardiovascular fitness quickly.

- **Illustration:** Set a timer for intervals of 30 seconds of work and 30 seconds of rest. Push yourself during the work intervals and recover during the rest periods.

Day 6: Active Recreation
- **Exercise:** Engage in active recreation such as playing sports, dancing, or hiking for 45 minutes.

- **Health Benefits:** Active recreation improves mood, builds endurance, and provides a fun way to stay active.

- **Illustration:** Gather friends or family members for a soccer game, put on your favorite playlist, dance around the house, or explore a local hiking trail.

Week 3: Maintaining Consistency
Day 7: Rest and Recovery

- **Exercise:** Take a rest day to allow your body to recover and recharge.

- **Health Benefits**: Rest days prevent burnout, reduce the risk of injury, and allow muscles to repair and grow.

- **Illustration:** Use this day to relax, practice mindfulness, and engage in activities that promote stress relief, such as meditation or gentle stretching.

Day 8: Swimming or Water Aerobics

- **Exercise:** Swim laps at your local pool or participate in a water aerobics class for 30 minutes.

- **Health Benefits:** Swimming strengthens muscles, improves cardiovascular health, and provides a low-impact workout.

- **Illustration:** Put on your swimsuit, goggles, and swim cap, and enjoy the refreshing sensation of moving through the water.

Day 9: Circuit Training

- **Exercise:** Complete a 45-minute circuit training workout involving strength exercises, cardio intervals, and flexibility movements.

- **Health Benefits:** Circuit training improves overall fitness, burns calories, and enhances muscular endurance.

- **Illustration:** Set up stations for different exercises (e.g., squats, jumping rope, yoga poses) and move from one station to the next with minimal rest between exercises.

CHAPTER 4: MENTAL HEALTH, SLEEP, AND PREDIABETES

Stress Management Techniques and Their Role in Blood Sugar Control

Many people consider stress a regular part of their everyday lives in today's fast-paced world. Stressors, which can range from demanding work demands to demanding family obligations, can be debilitating to our mental and physical well-being. Stress management strategies are essential for prediabetes management since they help to keep blood sugar levels at optimal ranges and promote general health.

Understanding Stress and Its Effects:

Stress is the body's natural response to perceived threats or challenges, triggering the release of stress hormones such as cortisol and adrenaline. While short-term stress can be helpful in certain situations, chronic or excessive stress can harm health. When we experience stress, our bodies go into "fight or flight" mode, increasing heart rate, blood pressure, and blood sugar levels to prepare for action.

The Link Between Stress and Blood Sugar:

Stress can significantly impact blood sugar levels, particularly for individuals with prediabetes or diabetes. When stress hormones are released, they signal the liver to produce more glucose, leading to high blood sugar levels. Additionally, stress can impair insulin sensitivity, making it more difficult for cells to respond to insulin and regulate blood sugar effectively. Over time, chronic stress can contribute to insulin resistance, a critical factor in the development of type 2 diabetes.

Effective Stress Management Techniques:

Managing stress is essential for maintaining optimal blood sugar control and overall health. Here are some effective stress management techniques:

- **Deep Breathing Exercises:** Deep breathing exercises, such as diaphragmatic breathing or the 4-7-8 technique, can activate the body's relaxation response, reduce stress hormones, and promote a sense of calmness and well-being.
- **Regular Exercise:** Regular physical activity, such as walking, jogging, or yoga, can help reduce stress levels, boost mood-enhancing endorphins, and improve insulin sensitivity.
- **Mindfulness Meditation:** Mindfulness meditation involves bringing awareness to the present moment without judgment. It can help reduce stress, promote emotional balance, and improve well-being.
- **Social Support:** Seeking support from friends, family, or support groups can provide a sense of connection, validation, and understanding during stress. Sharing your feelings and receiving encouragement from others can help alleviate stress and promote resilience.
- **Healthy Lifestyle Habits:** Healthy lifestyle habits, such as getting adequate sleep, eating a balanced diet, and limiting caffeine and alcohol intake, can help support overall stress management and blood sugar control.

Importance of Quality Sleep for Metabolic Health

Sleep is often undervalued in today's fast-paced society, yet it plays a crucial role in our overall health and well-being. Regarding metabolic health, quality sleep is essential for maintaining optimal blood sugar levels, supporting weight management, and reducing the risk of developing chronic diseases such as type 2 diabetes.

Understanding the Sleep Cycle:

Quality sleep involves cycling through different stages of sleep, including light sleep, deep sleep, and rapid eye movement (REM) sleep. Each stage uniquely supports physical and mental restoration, memory consolidation, and overall well-being. The sleep cycle typically repeats every 90 to 120 minutes, with REM sleep becoming longer and more frequent in the latter half of the night.

Impact of Sleep on Hormones:

Sleep plays a significant role in regulating hormones in appetite control, metabolism, and blood sugar. When we don't get enough sleep or experience poor sleep quality, our hormonal balance is disrupted, leading to increased hunger, decreased satiety, and impaired glucose metabolism. Here's how sleep influences critical hormones:

- **Leptin and Ghrelin:** Leptin, known as the "satiety hormone," signals feelings of fullness and helps regulate appetite, while ghrelin, known as the "hunger hormone," stimulates appetite and promotes food intake. Sleep deprivation disrupts the balance between leptin and ghrelin, leading to increased hunger and overeating.

- **Insulin:** Sleep deprivation can impair insulin sensitivity, making it more difficult for cells to respond to insulin and regulate blood sugar levels effectively. This can lead to insulin resistance, a precursor to type 2 diabetes and contribute to high blood sugar levels over time.

- **Cortisol:** Cortisol, often called the "stress hormone," regulates metabolism, blood sugar levels, and inflammation. Disrupted sleep patterns or chronic sleep deprivation can lead to dysregulation of cortisol levels, contributing to metabolic dysfunction and increased risk of diabetes.

Effects of Sleep Deprivation on Metabolic Health:

Chronic sleep deprivation or poor sleep quality has been linked to a range of metabolic health issues, including:

- **Weight Gain:** Lack of sleep disrupts the balance of hunger and satiety hormones, leading to increased appetite, cravings for high-calorie foods, and weight gain over time.

- **Insulin Resistance:** Sleep deprivation impairs insulin sensitivity, leading to high blood sugar levels and increased risk of insulin resistance, a critical factor in developing type 2 diabetes.

- **Increased Risk of Type 2 Diabetes:** Studies have shown that individuals who consistently experience poor sleep quality or short sleep duration are at an increased risk of developing type 2 diabetes compared to those who get an adequate amount of sleep.

Mindfulness Practices and Their Impact on Prediabetes

Introducing mindfulness practices into our daily lives can be a potent remedy to the stresses of modern living in our fast-paced society, where stressors and distractions are everywhere. Mindfulness activities are promising for people with prediabetes because they provide a comprehensive strategy for regulating their physical and emotional health.

Understanding Mindfulness:

Mindfulness is a state of heightened awareness and non-judgmental presence in the present moment. It involves intentionally paying attention to thoughts, feelings, bodily sensations, and the surrounding environment with curiosity and acceptance. Mindfulness practices stem from ancient contemplative traditions such as Buddhism but have gained widespread popularity in modern psychology and wellness circles for their therapeutic benefits.

Impact of Mindfulness on Prediabetes:

Mindfulness practices can positively influence various aspects of prediabetes management, including:

- **Stress Reduction:** Chronic stress is a common contributor to prediabetes and exacerbates insulin resistance. Mindfulness techniques such as meditation, deep breathing, and body scan exercises promote relaxation, reduce stress hormones like cortisol, and foster emotional resilience in life's challenges.
- **Blood Sugar Regulation:** Studies have shown that mindfulness practices can improve blood sugar control and reduce HbA1c levels in individuals with prediabetes. By cultivating mindfulness, individuals become more attuned to their body's signals, making healthier lifestyle choices, and responding more skillfully to cravings and emotional eating triggers.
- **Emotional Well-being:** Prediabetes diagnosis can trigger feelings of anxiety, fear, and uncertainty about the future. Mindfulness practices provide tools for managing difficult emotions, cultivating self-compassion, and fostering a sense of acceptance and stability in the face of adversity.
- **Healthy Eating Habits:** Mindful eating, a form of mindfulness applied to eating, encourages individuals to slow down, savor each bite, and pay attention to hunger and fullness cues. By practicing mindful eating, individuals with prediabetes can develop a more intuitive relationship with food, make healthier food choices, and avoid overeating.

Incorporating Mindfulness into Daily Life:

It takes little effort or specific training to incorporate mindfulness into daily living. Easy routines like walking, pausing, checking in with yourself throughout the day, and mindful breathing can significantly impact your general well-being. Moreover, advice and assistance in creating a regular mindfulness practice can be obtained by enrolling in mindfulness-based stress reduction (M.B.S.R.) courses or participating in structured mindfulness programs.

PART II: MEAL PLAN AND RECIPES

CHAPTER 5: CREATING A 3-WEEK PREDIABETES REVERSAL PLAN

Starting the process of reversing prediabetes requires a multifaceted strategy that includes dietary adjustments, exercise, and lifestyle modifications. Creating an organised meal plan that supports regulated blood sugar levels, encourages weight loss, and offers necessary nutrients is one of the most critical aspects of this trip. This chapter will walk you through putting together a three-week plan to reverse prediabetes, emphasising generating well-balanced meals and snacks. It also provides sample meal plans, helpful grocery shopping advice, and ingredient substitutions.

Designing Balanced Meals and Snacks

Creating balanced meals and snacks is crucial for managing blood sugar levels and preventing spikes and crashes. Here's how you can design meals that are both nutritious and delicious:

- **Carbohydrates:** Select complex carbs, including whole grains, legumes, and veggies with a low glycemic index. These carbohydrates digest slowly, providing a steady release of glucose into the bloodstream.
- **Proteins:** Include lean protein sources in every meal to help stabilize blood sugar levels. Examples include chicken, fish, tofu, legumes, and low-fat dairy products.
- **Fats:** Include heart-healthy fats from nuts, seeds, avocados, and olive oil. These fats help you feel full longer and can improve insulin sensitivity.
- **Fiber:** High-fiber foods are essential for slowing the absorption of sugar and promoting digestive health. Add plenty of fruits, veggies, whole grains, and legumes.
- **Portion Control:** Pay attention to portion sizes to avoid overeating. Using smaller plates and being mindful of serving sizes can help maintain balanced blood sugar levels.

- **Hydration:** Drink plenty of water throughout the day to stay hydrated and support overall metabolic function.

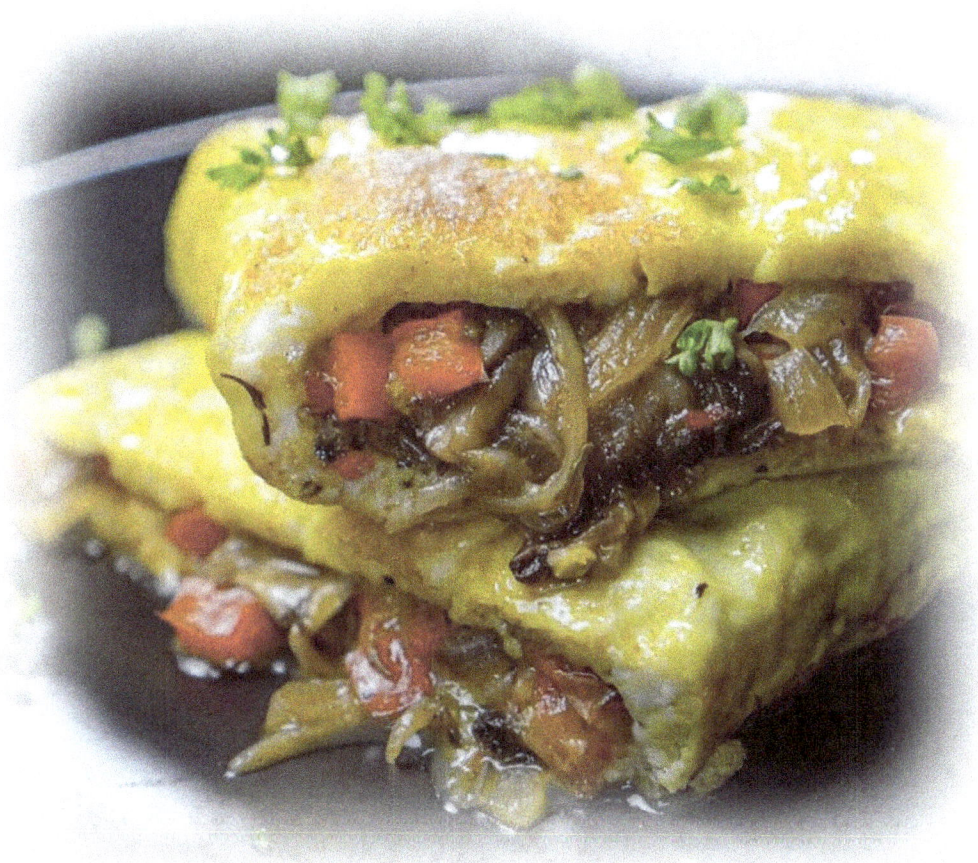

3 Weeks SAMPLE MEAL PLANS

Sample Meal Plans for Breakfast Lunch Dinner and Snacks

To help you get started, here are sample meal plans for each day of the week, ensuring variety and nutritional balance:

Week 1:

Day 1:

- **Breakfast:** Greek yoghurt with mixed berries and a sprinkle of chia seeds
- **Lunch:** Quinoa salad with grilled chicken, mixed greens, cherry tomatoes, and a lemon vinaigrette
- **Dinner:** Baked salmon with a side of roasted Brussels sprouts and sweet potato wedges
- **Snack:** Apple slices with almond butter

Day 2:

- **Breakfast:** Overnight oats with rolled oats, almond milk, sliced banana, and a dash of cinnamon
- **Lunch:** Len soup with a whole-grain roll and a side salad
- **Dinner:** Brown rice, bell peppers, and broccoli with stir-fried tofu
- **Snack:** Carrot sticks with hummus

Day 3:

- **Breakfast:** spinach, tomatoes, and mushrooms in a veggie omelet
- **Lunch:** Turkey and avocado wrapped in a whole-grain tortilla with a side of mixed greens
- **Dinner:** Grilled shrimp with quinoa and steamed asparagus
- **Snack:** A handful of mixed nuts

Week 2:

Day 1:

- **Breakfast:** Smoothie with spinach, frozen berries, protein powder, and almond milk
- **Lunch:** Chickpea and vegetable curry with a side of brown rice
- **Dinner:** Grilled chicken breast with a side of roasted vegetables and a quinoa salad
- **Snack:** Greek yoghurt with a drizzle of honey and chopped walnuts

Day 2:

- **Breakfast:** Avocado on whole-grain bread with a poached egg
- **Lunch:** Lime-dressed black bean and corn salad
- **Dinner:** Baked cod with a side of sautéed spinach and mashed cauliflower
- **Snack:** Sliced cucumber with tzatziki sauce

Day 3:

- **Breakfast:** pineapple pieces mixed with cottage cheese and topped with flaxseeds
- **Lunch:** Spinach and feta stuffed chicken breast with a side of quinoa
- **Dinner:** Marinara sauce-topped turkey meatballs with zucchini noodles
- **Snack:** Celery sticks with peanut butter

Week 3:

Day 1:

- **Breakfast:** Chia pudding made with chia seeds, almond milk, and a splash of vanilla extract
- **Lunch:** Tabbouleh salad with parsley, tomatoes, cucumbers, and bulgur
- **Dinner:** Grilled salmon with a side of quinoa and steamed broccoli.
- **Snack:** Berries with a dollop of Greek yoghurt

Day 2:

- **Breakfast:** Smoothie bowl with blended frozen berries, spinach, and almond milk, topped with granola
- **Lunch:** Bell peppers filled with veggies, black beans, and quinoa
- **Dinner:** Grilled tilapia with a side of wild rice and steamed broccoli
- **Snack:** Whole-grain crackers with cheese

Day 3:

- **Breakfast:** Banana pancakes made with mashed bananas, eggs, and a touch of oats
- **Lunch:** Mixed bean salad with kidney beans, chickpeas, and lentils, dressed with olive oil and lemon juice
- **Dinner:** Beef stir-fry with a variety of colorful vegetables and brown rice
- **Snack:** A little bowl filled with air-popped popcorn

NOTE:

" Reversing prediabetes involves a comprehensive approach that includes dietary adjustments, exercise, and lifestyle changes. One of the most important steps is creating an organized meal plan that helps regulate blood sugar levels, supports weight loss, and provides essential nutrients."

Grocery Shopping Tips and Ingredient Substitutions

Making a strategy before grocery shopping might help you stick to your prediabetes reversal objectives. To make your shopping trip effective, consider the following advice and ingredient substitutions:

Plan Ahead: Before heading to the store, list the ingredients for your meals and snacks. Planning your weekly meals can help you avoid impulse buys and ensure you have everything you need.

Shop the Perimeter: Most fresh produce, lean proteins, and dairy products are around the store's perimeter. Focus on these areas and avoid processed foods found in the Centre aisles.

Read Labels: When buying packaged foods, read the nutrition labels to check for added sugars, unhealthy fats, and artificial ingredients. Choose products with minimal ingredients and no added sugars.

Healthy Substitutions:

- **White rice:** Substitute with brown rice, quinoa, or cauliflower rice.
- **Pasta:** Use whole-grain pasta, zucchini noodles, or spaghetti squash.
- **Bread:** Opt for whole-grain bread or wraps instead of white bread.
- **Sugary snacks:** Replace with fresh fruit, nuts, or Greek yoghurt with berries.
- **Soda:** Choose sparkling water with a splash of fruit juice or herbal tea.
- **High-fat dairy:** Use low-fat or non-dairy alternatives like almond milk or Greek yoghurt.

Buy in Bulk: Purchasing whole grains, nuts, seeds, and legumes in bulk can save money and ensure you have healthy staples.

Fresh vs. Frozen: Fresh produce is great, but frozen fruits and vegetables can be just as nutritious and are convenient for quick meals. They also have a longer shelf life, reducing waste.

Seasonal Shopping: Buying seasonal produce can be cost-effective and ensure you get the freshest options. Farmers' markets are a great place to find seasonal and locally grown fruits and vegetables.

KEY IDEAS	

BREAKFASTS AND SMOOTHIES

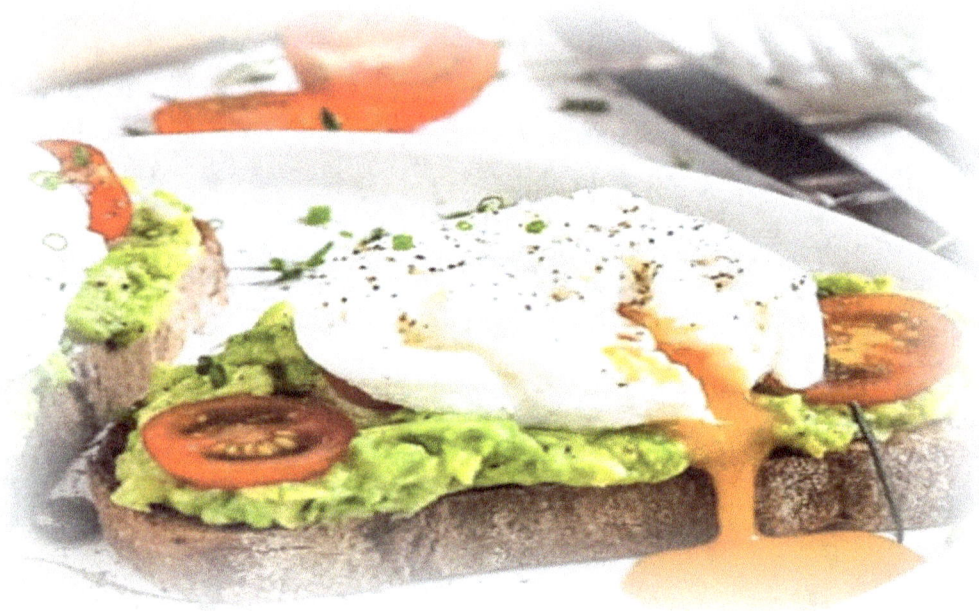

Eating a healthy breakfast early in the day establishes the foundation for stable blood sugar levels and long-lasting energy. People controlling their prediabetes need to make breakfast choices high in fiber, protein, and healthy fats while watching how much carbohydrates they eat. Many smoothie and breakfast dishes in this chapter are designed to help regulate blood sugar. Food prep suggestions are also given to help you stay on schedule on hectic mornings. We will also highlight some smoothie and breakfast options that should be avoided since they may harm blood sugar levels.

NUTRIENT-DENSE BREAKFAST OPTIONS FOR BLOOD SUGAR CONTROL

Veggie Omelet with Spinach, Tomatoes, and Mushrooms

- **Carb Count:** 5g
- **Nutritional Value Count and Balance**: 200 calories, 14g protein, 10g fat, 5g carbs
- **Serving Size:** 1 omelet
- **Prep Time:** 15 minutes

Ingredients:
- two large eggs
- 1/4 cup spinach, chopped
- 1/4 cup cherry tomatoes, halved
- 1/4 cup mushrooms, sliced
- 1 tbsp olive oil
- Salt and pepper to taste

Directions:
- In a nonstick pan, warm the olive oil over medium heat.
- Add mushrooms and tomatoes and sauté for 3-4 minutes.
- Add spinach and cook until wilted.
- Whisk eggs in a bowl, pour over the veggies, and cook until set.
- Season with salt and pepper.

Health Benefit: Provides high-quality protein and fiber, stabilising blood sugar and satiety.

Overnight Oats with Chia Seeds and Berries

- **Carb Count:** 35g
- **Nutritional Value Count and Balance:** 250 calories, 8g protein, 7g fat, 35g carbs, 8g fiber
- **Serving Size:** 1 jar
- **Prep Time**: 10 minutes (plus freezing overnight)

Ingredients:
- 1/2 cup rolled oats
- 1 tbsp chia seeds
- 1/2 cup unsweetened almond milk
- 1/4 cup mixed berries
- 1 tsp honey (optional)

Directions:
- Combine oats, chia seeds, and almond milk in a jar.
- Stir well and refrigerate overnight.
- Top with berries and honey before serving.

Health Benefit: High in fiber and antioxidants, promoting digestive health and reducing inflammation.

Greek Yogurt Parfait with Nuts and Berries

- **Carb Count:** 20g
- **Nutritional Value Count and Balance:** 220 calories, 15g protein, 9g fat, 20g carbs
- **Serving Size**: 1 parfait
- **Prep Time:** 5 minutes

Ingredients:
- 1 cup Greek yogurt
- 1/4 cup mixed berries
- 2 tbsp chopped nuts (almonds, walnuts)
- 1 tsp flax seeds

Directions:
- Layer Greek yoghurt, berries, and nuts in a glass bowl.
- Sprinkle with flax seeds.

Health Benefit: Rich in protein, healthy fats, and probiotics for gut health and blood sugar control.

Avocado Toast with Whole Grain Bread

- **Carb Count:** 30g
- **Nutritional Value Count and Balance:** 280 calories, 6g protein, 20g fat, 30g carbs, 10g fiber
- **Serving Size:** 1 toast
- **Prep Time:** 5 minutes

Ingredients:
- one slice whole grain bread
- 1/2 avocado
- 1 tsp lemon juice
- Salt and pepper to taste

Directions:
- Toast the bread.
- Add the lemon juice, salt, and pepper and mash the avocado.
- Spread the avocado mixture on the toast.

Health Benefit: Healthy fats from avocado help maintain steady blood sugar levels.

Cottage Cheese with Pineapple and Flaxseeds

- **Carb Count:** 15g
- **Nutritional Value Count and Balance**: 180 calories, 14g protein, 5g fat, 15g carbs
- **Serving Size:** 1 bowl
- **Prep Time:** 5 minutes

Ingredients:
- 1 cup cottage cheese
- 1/4 cup pineapple chunks
- 1 tsp flaxseeds

Directions:
- In a bowl, mix cottage cheese and pineapple.
- Sprinkle with flaxseeds.

Health Benefit: High in protein and fiber, promoting satiety and stable blood sugar levels.

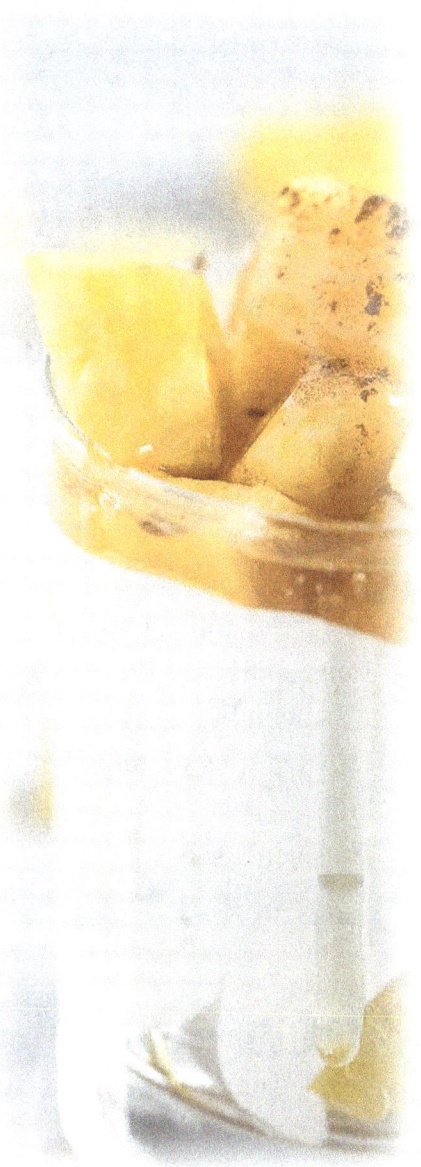

Energizing Smoothie Recipes For Prediabetes Management

Green Apple Smoothie

- **Carb Count:** 25g
- **Nutritional Value Count and Balance:** 150 calories, 5g protein, 2g fat, 25g carbs
- **Serving Size:** 1 glass
- **Prep Time:** 5 minutes

Ingredients:
- one green apple, chopped
- 1 cup spinach
- 1/2 cucumber
- 1/2 cup unsweetened almond milk
- 1 tbsp chia seeds

Directions:
- Blend all ingredients until smooth.

Health Benefit: Rich in fiber and antioxidants, supporting blood sugar control and hydration.

Berry Protein Smoothie

Carb Count: 20g
Nutritional Value Count and Balance: 200 calories, 15g protein, 5g fat, 20g carbs
Serving Size: 1 glass
Prep Time: 5 minutes

Ingredients:
- 1/2 cup mixed berries
- one scoop of protein powder
- 1/2 banana
- 1 cup unsweetened almond milk
- 1 tbsp flaxseeds

Directions:
- Blend all ingredients until smooth.

Health Benefit: High in protein and fiber, aiding in muscle recovery and blood sugar management.

Tropical Mango Smoothie

- **Carb Count:** 30g
- **Nutritional Value Count and Balance:** 180 calories, 4g protein, 2g fat, 30g carbs
- **Serving Size:** 1 glass
- **Prep Time:** 5 minutes

Ingredients:
- 1/2 cup mango chunks
- 1/2 cup pineapple chunks
- 1/2 banana
- 1 cup coconut water

Directions:
- Blend all ingredients until smooth.

Health Benefit: Rich in vitamins and electrolytes, promoting hydration and energy.

Peanut Butter Banana Smoothie

- **Carb Count:** 35g
- **Nutritional Value Count and Balance:** 250 calories, 8g protein, 10g fat, 35g carbs
- **Serving Size:** 1 glass
- **Prep Time:** 5 minutes

Ingredients:
- one banana
- 1 tbsp peanut butter
- 1/2 cup Greek yogurt
- 1 cup unsweetened almond milk

Directions:
- Blend all ingredients until smooth.

Health Benefit: High in protein and healthy fats, providing sustained energy.

Detoxifying Green Smoothie

- **Carb Count:** 20g
- **Nutritional Value Count and Balance**: 130 calories, 4g protein, 2g fat, 20g carbs
- **Serving Size:** 1 glass
- **Prep Time:** 5 minutes

Ingredients:
- 1 cup kale
- 1/2 cucumber
- one green apple
- 1 tbsp lemon juice
- 1 cup water

Directions:
- Blend all ingredients until smooth.

Health Benefit: Packed with detoxifying greens and antioxidants, supporting overall health.

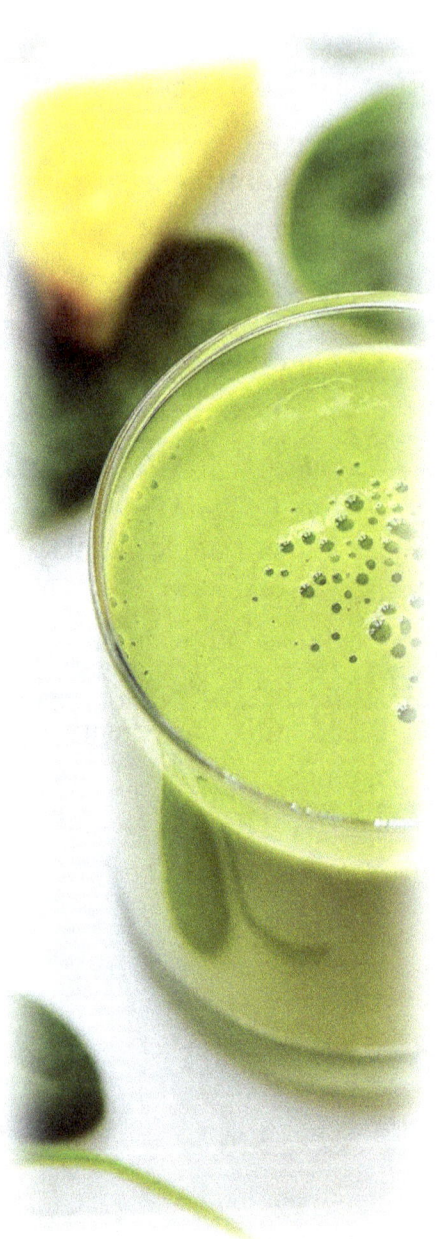

Meal Prep Tips for Busy Mornings

Batch Cooking: At the beginning of the week, prepare large quantities of breakfast items like overnight oats or chia pudding. Store them in individual portions for quick grab-and-go options.

Pre-Chopped Ingredients: Chop vegetables and fruits ahead of time and store them in airtight containers. This reduces prep time in the morning.

Smoothie Packs: Prepare smoothie packs by placing all the ingredients (except the liquid) in zip-lock bags and freezing them. In the morning, add the liquid and blend.

Mason Jar Meals: Layer ingredients in mason jars for parfaits or salads. These jars keep the ingredients fresh and can be easily transported.

Set a Routine: Establish a morning routine that includes time for a healthy breakfast. Consistency helps reinforce good habits and ensures you start your day right.

Avoided Breakfasts and Smoothies:

1. Sugary Cereals:
- **Why to Avoid:** High in added sugars and refined carbs, leading to blood sugar spikes and crashes.

2. Flavored Yogurts:
- **Why to Avoid:** It often contains high amounts of added sugars, negating the health benefits of yoghurt.

3. Pastries and Doughnuts:
- **Why to Avoid:** High in refined sugars and unhealthy fats, causing rapid blood sugar spikes and weight gain.

4. Fruit Juices:
- **Why to Avoid**: Lack of fiber and are high in natural sugars, leading to quick absorption and blood sugar spikes.

5. Sweetened Smoothies:
- **Why to Avoid:** Pre-made or store-bought smoothies can be high in added sugars and calorics, impacting blood sugar levels negatively.

SALADS AND LIGHT MAINS

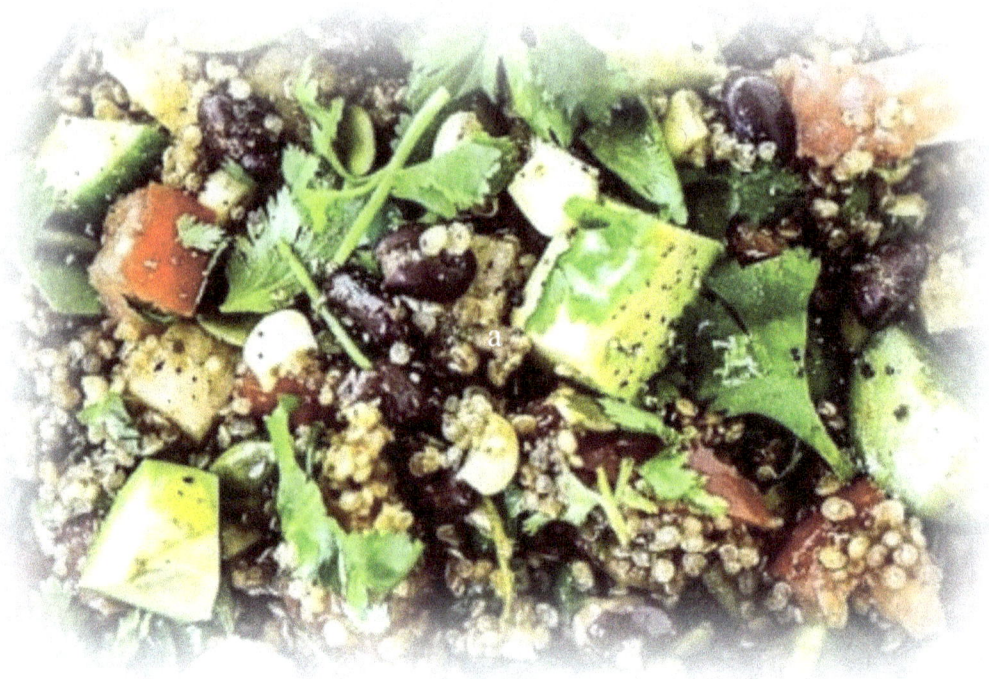

Eating healthily doesn't require labor-intensive cooking or sophisticated recipes. The nutrients and flavors you need to maintain your health, especially when managing prediabetes, can be found in salads and light main dishes. With an eye on reducing carbohydrate intake, this section provides a selection of salads and light main dishes high in fiber, protein, and healthy fats. Every recipe has comprehensive nutritional data and helpful hints to make preparation a breeze. We'll also highlight a few popular salads and light main options you should avoid because they might raise your blood sugar levels.

Wholesome Salad Recipes Packed with Fiber and Flavor

Mediterranean Chickpea Salad

- **Carb Count:** 30g
- **Nutritional Value Count and Balance:** 280 calories, 8g protein, 12g fat, 30g carbs, 8g fiber
- **Serving Size:** 1 bowl
- **Prep Time:** 15 minutes

Ingredients:
- 1 can chickpeas, rinsed and drained
- 1 cucumber, diced
- 1/2 red bell pepper, diced
- 1/4 cup red onion, diced
- 1/4 cup Kalamata olives, sliced
- 2 tbsp feta cheese, crumbled
- 2 tbsp olive oil
- 1 tbsp red wine vinegar
- Salt and pepper to taste

Directions:
- Combine chickpeas, cucumber, red bell pepper, red onion, olives, and feta cheese in a large bowl.
- Drizzle with olive oil and red wine vinegar.
- Add salt and pepper to taste, then toss to mix.

Health Benefit: Rich in fiber and healthy fats, this salad supports heart health and helps control blood sugar levels.

Asian-Inspired Shrimp Salad

- **Carb Count:** 15g
- **Nutritional Value Count and Balance:** 200 calories, 18g protein, 7g fat, 15g carbs
- **Serving Size:** 1 plate
- **Prep Time:** 20 minutes

Ingredients:
- 12 shrimp, cooked and peeled
- 2 cups mixed greens
- 1/2 cup shredded carrots
- 1/2 cup red bell pepper, sliced
- 1/4 cup green onions, chopped
- 2 tbsp sesame oil
- 1 tbsp soy sauce (low sodium)
- 1 tbsp rice vinegar

Directions:
- In a large bowl, combine shrimp, mixed greens, carrots, bell pepper, and green onions.
- Drizzle with sesame oil, soy sauce, and rice vinegar.
- Toss to combine.

Health Benefit: This salad is high in protein and antioxidants and helps boost immunity and maintain healthy blood sugar levels.

Quinoa and Black Bean Salaz

- **Carb Count:** 35g
- **Nutritional Value Count and Balance:** 300 calories, 10g protein, 8g fat, 35g carbs, 7g fiber
- **Serving Size:** 1 bowl
- **Prep Time:** 20 minutes

Ingredients:

- 1 cup cooked quinoa
- 1 cup black beans, rinsed and drained
- 1/2 cup corn kernels
- 1/2 cup cherry tomatoes, halved
- 1/4 cup red onion, diced
- 1 avocado, diced
- 2 tbsp olive oil
- 1 tbsp lime juice
- Salt and pepper to taste

Directions:

- In a large bowl, combine quinoa, black beans, corn, tomatoes, red onion, and avocado.
- Pour in some lime juice and olive oil.
- Add salt and pepper to taste, then toss to mix.

Health Benefit: High in fiber and plant-based protein, this salad supports digestive health and helps maintain stable blood sugar levels.

Grilled Chicken Caesar Salad

- **Carb Count:** 10g
- **Nutritional Value Count and Balance:** 350 calories, 30g protein, 20g fat, 10g carbs
- **Serving Size:** 1 plate
- **Prep Time:** 25 minutes

Ingredients:

- 1 grilled chicken breast, sliced
- 4 cups romaine lettuce, chopped
- 1/4 cup grated Parmesan cheese
- 1/2 cup cherry tomatoes, halved
- 2 tbsp Caesar dressing (preferably low-fat)

Directions:

- Combine lettuce, chicken, Parmesan cheese, and cherry tomatoes in a large bowl.
- Drizzle with Caesar dressing and toss to combine.

Health Benefit: Packed with lean protein and vitamins, this salad is perfect for a balanced, low-carb meal.

Avocado and Tuna Salad

- **Carb Count:** 12g
- **Nutritional Value Count and Balance**: 250 calories, 20g protein, 15g fat, 12g carbs
- **Serving Size:** 1 bowl
- **Prep Time:** 10 minutes

Ingredients:

- 1 can tuna in water, drained
- 1 avocado, diced
- 1/2 cup cherry tomatoes, halved
- 1/4 cup red onion, diced
- 2 tbsp olive oil
- 1 tbsp lemon juice
- Salt and pepper to taste

Directions:

- In a large bowl, combine tuna, avocado, cherry tomatoes, and red onion.
- Pour in some lemon juice and olive oil.
- Add salt and pepper to taste, then toss to mix.

Health Benefit: This salad contains healthy fats and protein and helps control weight and blood sugar.

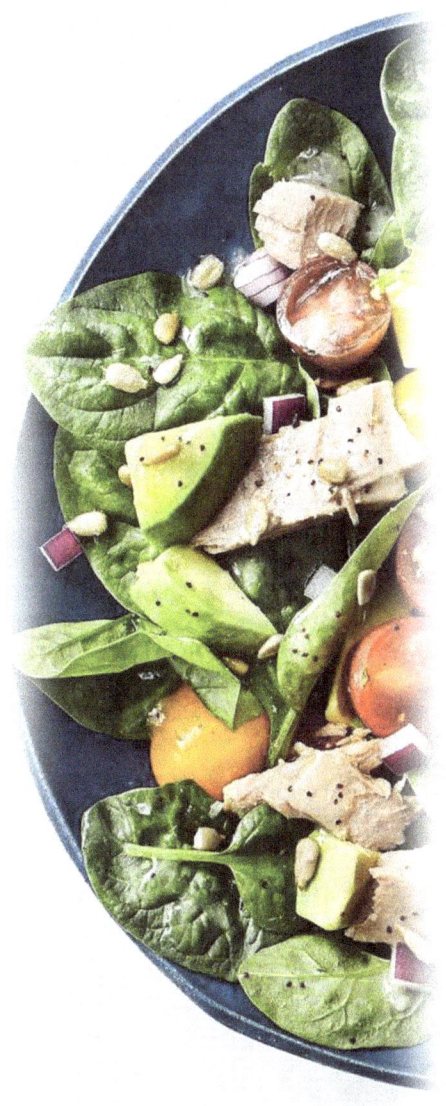

Turkey and Avocado Wrap

- **Carb Count:** 25g
- **Nutritional Value Count and Balance:** 350 calories, 25g protein, 15g fat, 25g carbs
- **Serving Size:** 1 wrap
- **Prep Time:** 10 minutes

Ingredients:
- 1 whole wheat tortilla
- 3 slices turkey breast
- 1/2 avocado, sliced
- 1/4 cup mixed greens
- 1 tbsp hummus

Directions:
- Spread hummus on the tortilla.
- Layer turkey, avocado, and mixed greens.
- Roll up the tortilla and cut it in half.

Health Benefit: Provides a balanced mix of protein, healthy fats, and fiber, supporting sustained energy.

Lentil and Veggie Bowl

- **Carb Count:** 40g
- **Nutritional Value Count and Balance:** 320 calories, 12g protein, 10g fat, 40g carbs
- **Serving Size:** 1 bowl
- **Prep Time:** 20 minutes

Ingredients:
- 1 cup cooked lentils
- 1/2 cup roasted sweet potatoes
- 1/2 cup steamed broccoli
- 1/4 cup diced red bell pepper
- 2 tbsp tahini sauce

Directions:
- In a bowl, combine lentils, sweet potatoes, broccoli, and red bell pepper.
- Drizzle with tahini sauce and mix well.

Health Benefit: High in fiber and plant-based protein, supporting digestive health and blood sugar regulation.

Salmon and Quinoa Bowl

- **Carb Count:** 35g
- **Nutritional Value Count and Balance:** 400 calories, 30g protein, 15g fat, 35g carbs
- **Serving Size:** 1 bowl
- **Prep Time:** 25 minutes

Ingredients:
- 1 salmon fillet, grilled
- 1 cup cooked quinoa
- 1/2 cup steamed asparagus
- 1/4 cup cherry tomatoes, halved
- 2 tbsp olive oil
- 1 tbsp lemon juice

Directions:
- In a bowl, combine quinoa, asparagus, and cherry tomatoes.
- Top with grilled salmon.
- Pour in some lemon juice and olive oil.

Health Benefit: Rich in omega-3 fatty acids and protein, promoting heart health and stable blood sugar levels.

Chicken and Veggie Stir-Fry

- **Carb Count:** 20g
- **Nutritional Value Count and Balance:** 300 calories, 25g protein, 10g fat, 20g carbs
- **Serving Size:** 1 plate
- **Prep Time:** 20 minutes

Ingredients:
- 1 chicken breast, sliced
- 1 cup mixed bell peppers, sliced
- 1/2 cup snap peas
- 1/4 cup onions, sliced
- 2 tbsp soy sauce (low sodium)
- 1 tbsp sesame oil

Directions:
- Heat sesame oil in a pan over medium heat.
- Add chicken and cook until browned.
- Add vegetables and stir-fry until tender.
- Drizzle with soy sauce and mix well.

Health Benefit: High in protein and low in carbs, this stir-fry supports muscle health and stable blood sugar.

Eggplant and Chickpea Stew

- **Carb Count:** 35g
- **Nutritional Value Count and Balance:** 280 calories, 10g protein, 8g fat, 35g carbs, 10g fiber
- **Serving Size:** 1 bowl
- **Prep Time:** 30 minutes

Ingredients:

- 1 eggplant, diced
- 1 can chickpeas, rinsed and drained
- 1 cup diced tomatoes
- 1/2 cup onions, diced
- 2 cloves garlic, minced
- 2 tbsp olive oil
- 1 tsp cumin

Directions:

- In a pot, warm the olive oil over medium heat.
- Add the garlic and onions, and cook until tender.
- Add eggplant and cook until tender.
- Add chickpeas, tomatoes, and cumin. Simmer for 20 minutes.

Health Benefit: Packed with fiber and antioxidants, this stew supports digestive health and helps control blood sugar.

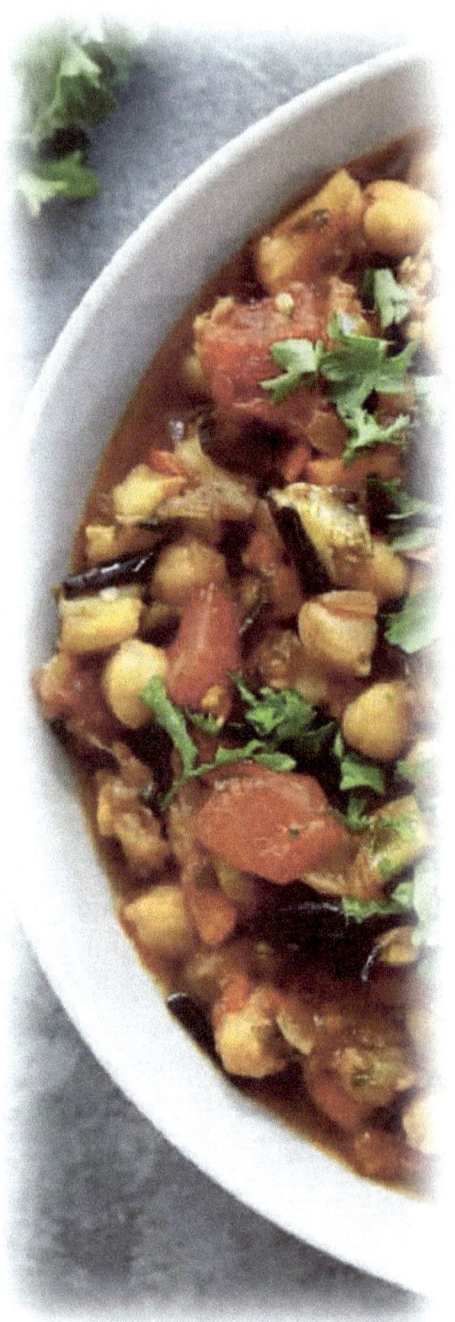

Quick and Easy Meal Solutions for Busy Weeknights

Stir-fried tofu and Vegetables

- **Carb Count:** 20g
- **Nutritional Value Count and Balance**: 250 calories, 15g protein, 12g fat, 20g carbs
- **Serving Size:** 1 plate
- **Prep Time:** 15 minutes

Ingredients:
- 1 cup tofu, cubed
- 1 cup mixed vegetables (broccoli, bell peppers, carrots)
- 2 tbsp soy sauce (low sodium)
- 1 tbsp sesame oil

Directions:
- On medium heat, warm up some sesame oil in a pan. Add tofu and cook until golden.
- Add vegetables and stir-fry until tender.
- Pour in the soy sauce and stir thoroughly.

Health Benefit: High in plant-based protein and low in carbs, supporting muscle health and stable blood sugar.

Zucchini Noodles with Pesto and Cherry Tomatoes

- **Carb Count:** 15g
- **Nutritional Value Count and Balance:** 220 calories, 10g protein, 15g fat, 15g carbs
- **Serving Size:** 1 plate
- **Prep Time**: 15 minutes

Ingredients:
- 2 medium zucchinis, spiralized
- 1/2 cup cherry tomatoes, halved
- 2 tbsp pesto

Directions:
- Sauté zucchini noodles in a big pan until they become soft.
- Add cherry tomatoes and cook for 2-3 minutes.
- Stir in pesto and mix well.

Health Benefit: Low in carbs and high in antioxidants, this dish supports weight management and stable blood sugar.

Greek Yogurt Chicken Salad

- **Carb Count:** 15g
- **Nutritional Value Count and Balance:** 300 calories, 25g protein, 10g fat, 15g carbs
- **Serving Size:** 1 plate
- **Prep Time:** 10 minutes

Ingredients:
- 1 chicken breast, cooked and diced
- 1/2 cup Greek yogurt
- 1/4 cup diced celery
- 1/4 cup grapes, halved
- 1 tbsp lemon juice

Directions:
- Combine chicken, Greek yoghurt, celery, grapes, and lemon juice in a bowl.
- Mix well and serve chilled.

Health Benefit: High in protein and probiotics, promoting gut health and stable blood sugar.

Stuffed Bell Peppers

- **Carb Count:** 30g
- **Nutritional Value Count and Balance:** 320 calories, 20g protein, 12g fat, 30g carbs
- **Serving Size:** 1 pepper
- **Prep Time:** 30 minutes

Ingredients:
- 4 bell peppers, cut off the tops and seeded
- 1 cup cooked quinoa
- 1/2 cup black beans
- 1/2 cup corn
- 1/4 cup diced tomatoes
- 1/4 cup shredded cheese

Directions:
- Preheat oven to 375°F.
- Mix a bowl of quinoa, black beans, corn, and tomatoes.
- Stuff each bell pepper with the mixture and top with cheese.
- Bake for 20 minutes.

Health Benefit: Rich in fiber and protein, supporting digestive health and stable blood sugar.

Spaghetti Squash with Marinara Sauce

- **Carb Count:** 25g
- **Nutritional Value Count and Balance:** 200 calories, 5g protein, 10g fat, 25g carbs
- **Serving Size:** 1 bowl
- **Prep Time:** 40 minutes

Ingredients:
- 1 spaghetti squash
- 1 cup marinara sauce
- 1/4 cup grated Parmesan cheese

Directions:
- Preheat oven to 375°F.
- After slicing the spaghetti squash in half, extract the seeds.
- Place the cut side on a baking sheet and bake for 35 to 40 minutes.
- Scrape out the flesh with a fork into strands.
- Add some Parmesan cheese and marinara sauce over top.

Health Benefit: Low in carbs and calories, supporting weight management, and stable blood sugar.

Avoided Salads and Light Mains

Caesar Salad with Croutons and Heavy Dressing
- **Why to Avoid:** High in unhealthy fats and refined carbs, leading to blood sugar spikes and increased calorie intake.

Macaroni Salad
- **Why to Avoid:** Made with refined pasta and mayonnaise, high in carbs and unhealthy fats, contributing to blood sugar spikes.

Breaded and Fried Chicken Salad
- **Why to Avoid:** High in unhealthy fats and carbs due to breading and frying, leading to poor blood sugar control.

Loaded Baked Potato with Bacon and Cheese
- **Why to Avoid**: High in carbs and saturated fats, causing rapid blood sugar spikes and weight gain.

Sweet and Sour Chicken
- **Why to Avoid:** High in sugar and refined carbs, leading to blood sugar spikes and increased calorie consumption.

HEARTY MAINS

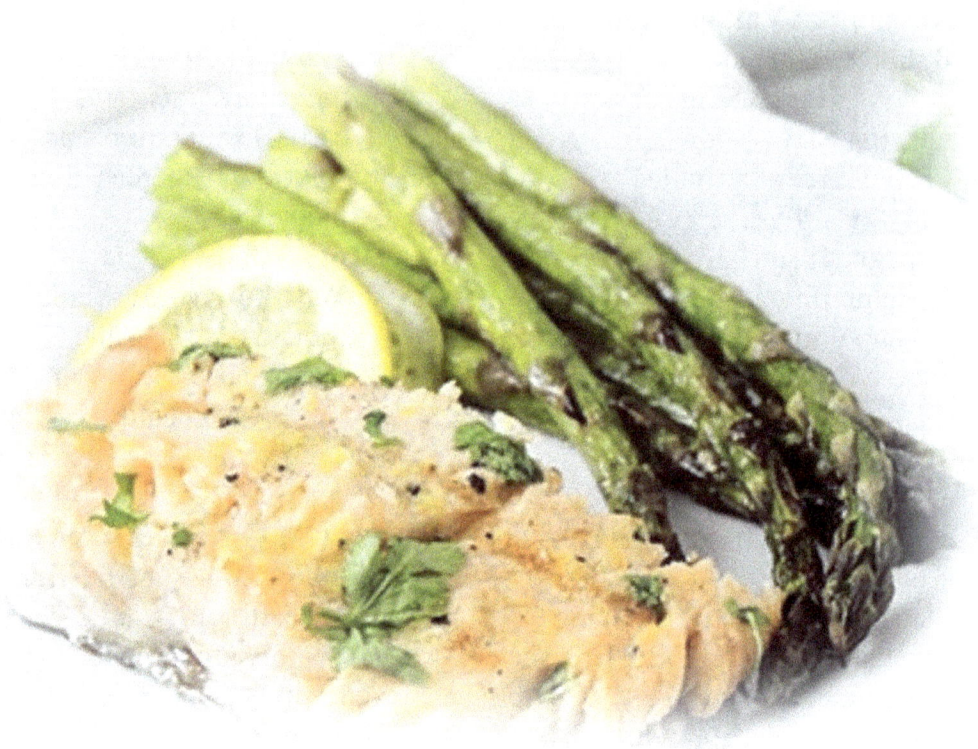

A healthy and filling dinner prevents prediabetes, preserves stable blood sugar levels, and improves overall health. This chapter includes a range of hearty main dishes that balance the needs for protein, healthy fats, and carbohydrates. Each recipe is designed to provide a satisfying dinner without compromising on nutrition. We'll also examine how to cook food to enhance flavor without compromising its health advantages. We'll also mention a few substantial main courses you should avoid due to the possibility of raising blood sugar.

Protein Rich Dinner Recipes for Prediabetes Reversal

Grilled Salmon with Asparagus

- **Carb Count:** 8g
- **Nutritional Value Count and Balance:** 350 calories, 30g protein, 22g fat, 8g carbs
- **Serving Size:** 1 plate
- **Prep Time:** 25 minutes

Ingredients:
- 1 salmon fillet
- 10 asparagus spears
- 1 tbsp olive oil
- 1 lemon (zested and juiced)
- Salt and pepper to taste

Directions:
- Preheat grill to medium-high heat.
- Drizzle salmon and asparagus with olive oil and season with salt, pepper, and lemon zest.
- Grill salmon on each side for 4-5 minutes until fully cooked.
- Grill asparagus for 3-4 minutes, turning frequently.
- Serve with a squeeze of lemon juice.

Health Benefit: High in omega-3 fatty acids and protein, supporting heart health and stable blood sugar levels.

Baked Chicken Breast with Quinoa and Spinach

- **Carb Count:** 30g
- **Nutritional Value Count and Balance:** 400 calories, 35g protein, 15g fat, 30g carbs
- **Serving Size:** 1 plate
- **Prep Time:** 35 minutes

Ingredients:
- 1 chicken breast
- 1 cup cooked quinoa
- 2 cups spinach
- 2 tbsp olive oil
- 1 garlic clove, minced
- Salt and pepper to taste

Directions:
- Preheat oven to 375°F.
- Season chicken with salt, pepper, and minced garlic.
- Place chicken in a baking dish and drizzle with olive oil.
- Bake for 25-30 minutes until fully cooked.
- Sauté spinach in a pan with a bit of olive oil until wilted.
- Serve chicken with quinoa and spinach.

Health Benefit: Provides a balanced mix of protein, fiber, and healthy fats, supporting muscle health and blood sugar control.

Beef and Broccoli Stir-Fry

- **Carb Count:** 20g
- **Nutritional Value Count and Balance:** 350 calories, 30g protein, 15g fat, 20g carbs
- **Serving Size:** 1 plate
- **Prep Time:** 20 minutes

Ingredients:
- 1 cup lean beef, sliced
- 2 cups broccoli florets
- 1/4 cup soy sauce (low sodium)
- 1 tbsp sesame oil
- 2 cloves garlic, minced

Directions:
- Heat sesame oil in a pan over medium-high heat.
- Add garlic and sauté until fragrant.
- Add beef and cook until browned.
- Add broccoli and soy sauce, and stir-fry until broccoli is tender.

Health Benefit: High in protein and antioxidants, supporting muscle repair and blood sugar stability.

Turkey Meatballs with Zucchini Noodles

- **Carb Count:** 15g
- **Nutritional Value Count and Balance:** 300 calories, 25g protein, 12g fat, 15g carbs
- **Serving Size:** 1 plate
- **Prep Time:** 30 minutes

Ingredients:
- 1 lb ground turkey
- 1 egg
- 1/4 cup almond flour
- 1/4 cup Parmesan cheese, grated
- 2 medium zucchinis, spiralized
- 1 cup marinara sauce (low sugar)

Directions:
- Preheat oven to 375°F.
- Mix ground turkey, egg, almond flour, and Parmesan cheese in a bowl.
- Form mixture into meatballs and place on a baking sheet.
- Bake for 20 minutes until fully cooked.
- Sauté zucchini noodles in a pan until tender.
- Serve meatballs over zucchini noodles with marinara sauce.

Health Benefit: Low in carbs and high in protein, supporting weight management and stable blood sugar levels.

Chicken Breast with Sweet Potato Mash

- **Carb Count:** 30g
- **Nutritional Value Count and Balance:** 400 calories, 35g protein, 12g fat, 30g carbs
- **Serving Size:** 1 plate
- **Prep Time:** 40 minutes

Ingredients:
- 1 large chicken breast
- 2 sweet potatoes, peeled and cubed
- 2 tbsp olive oil
- 1 tbsp rosemary, chopped
- Salt and pepper to taste

Directions:
- Preheat oven to 375°F (190°C).
- Season the chicken breast with rosemary, salt, and pepper.
- Heat 1 tablespoon of olive oil in an oven-safe pan over medium-high heat. Sear the chicken breast on both sides until golden brown, about 3-4 minutes per side.
- Transfer the pan to the preheated oven and bake for 20-25 minutes, or until the internal temperature of the chicken reaches 165°F (75°C).
- While baking the chicken, place the sweet potatoes in a large pot of boiling water. Cook until tender, about 15-20 minutes.
- Drain the sweet potatoes and mash them with 1 tablespoon olive oil. Season with salt and pepper to taste.
- Serve the baked chicken breast with the sweet potato mash.

Health Benefit: High in protein and complex carbs, this meal supports muscle health and provides sustained energy levels.

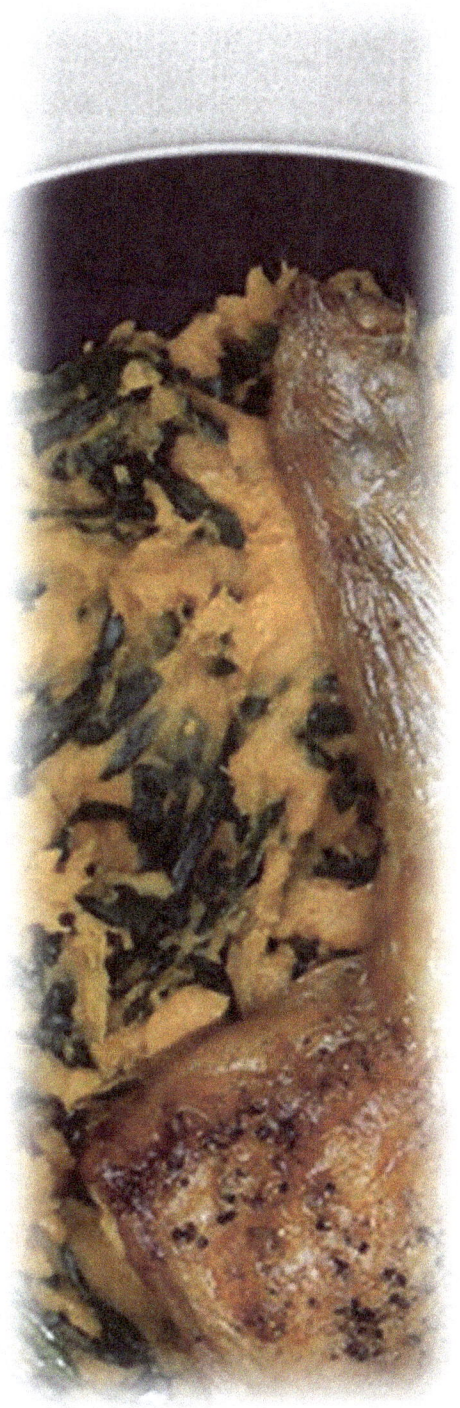

Vegetarian and Plant Based Options for Heart Health

Lentil and Vegetable Stew

- **Carb Count:** 40g
- **Nutritional Value Count and Balance**: 350 calories, 15g protein, 8g fat, 40g carbs, 12g fiber
- **Serving Size:** 1 bowl
- **Prep Time:** 30 minutes

Ingredients:
- 1 cup lentils
- 1 cup diced tomatoes
- 1 carrot, diced
- 1 celery stalk, diced
- 1 onion, chopped
- 2 cloves garlic, minced
- 4 cups vegetable broth
- 1 tbsp olive oil

Directions:
- Heat olive oil in a pot over medium heat.
- Add onion, garlic, carrot, celery, and sauté until soft.
- Add lentils, tomatoes, and broth.
- Simmer for 20 minutes until lentils are tender.

Health Benefit: High in fiber and plant-based protein, supporting heart health and blood sugar control.

Chickpea and Spinach Curry

- Carb Count: 35g
- Nutritional Value Count and Balance: 300 calories, 12g protein, 10g fat, 35g carbs
- Serving Size: 1 bowl
- Prep Time: 25 minutes

Ingredients:
- 1 can chickpeas, rinsed and drained
- 2 cups spinach
- 1 cup diced tomatoes
- 1 onion, chopped
- 2 cloves garlic, minced
- 1 tbsp curry powder
- 1 tbsp coconut oil

Directions:
- Heat coconut oil in a pot over medium heat.
- Add onion and garlic, and sauté until soft.
- Add chickpeas, tomatoes, curry powder, and spinach.
- Simmer for 15 minutes.

Health Benefit: Rich in fiber, antioxidants, and plant-based protein, supporting heart health and stable blood sugar levels.

Stuffed Bell Peppers with Quinoa and Black Beans

- **Carb Count:** 40g
- **Nutritional Value Count and Balance:** 350 calories, 15g protein, 10g fat, 40g carbs, 10g fiber
- Serving **Size:** 1 bell pepper
- **Prep Time:** 35 minutes

Ingredients:
- 4 bell peppers, tops removed and seeded
- 1 cup cooked quinoa
- 1 cup black beans, rinsed and drained
- 1/2 cup corn
- 1/2 cup diced tomatoes
- 1 tsp cumin

Directions:
- Preheat oven to 375°F.
- Mix quinoa, black beans, corn, tomatoes, and cumin bowl.
- Stuff bell peppers with the mixture.
- Bake for 25-30 minutes.

Health Benefit: High in fiber and plant-based protein, supporting digestive health and blood sugar control.

Mushroom and Barley Risotto

- **Carb Count:** 45g
- **Nutritional Value Count and Balance**: 350 calories, 12g protein, 10g fat, 45g carbs, 8g fiber
- **Serving Size:** 1 bowl
- **Prep Time:** 40 minutes

Ingredients:
- 1 cup pearl barley
- 2 cups mushrooms, sliced
- 1 onion, chopped
- 2 cloves garlic, minced
- 4 cups vegetable broth
- 1 tbsp olive oil

Directions:
- Heat olive oil in a pot over medium heat.
- Add onion, garlic, and mushrooms, and sauté until soft.
- Add barley and cook for 2-3 minutes.
- Gradually add broth, stirring frequently until barley is tender.

Health Benefit: High in fiber and complex carbs, supporting digestive health and sustained energy levels.

Eggplant Parmesan

- **Carb Count:** 30g
- **Nutritional Value Count and Balance:** 300 calories, 12g protein, 15g fat, 30g carbs
- **Serving Size:** 1 plate
- **Prep Time:** 45 minutes

Ingredients:
- 1 eggplant, sliced
- 1 cup marinara sauce
- 1/2 cup mozzarella cheese, shredded
- 1/4 cup Parmesan cheese, grated
- 1/4 cup almond flour

Directions:
- Preheat oven to 375°F.
- Dip eggplant slices in almond flour.
- Arrange in a baking dish and top with marinara sauce and cheese.
- Bake for 30-35 minutes.

Health Benefit: Low in carbs and high in antioxidants, supporting heart health and stable blood sugar levels.

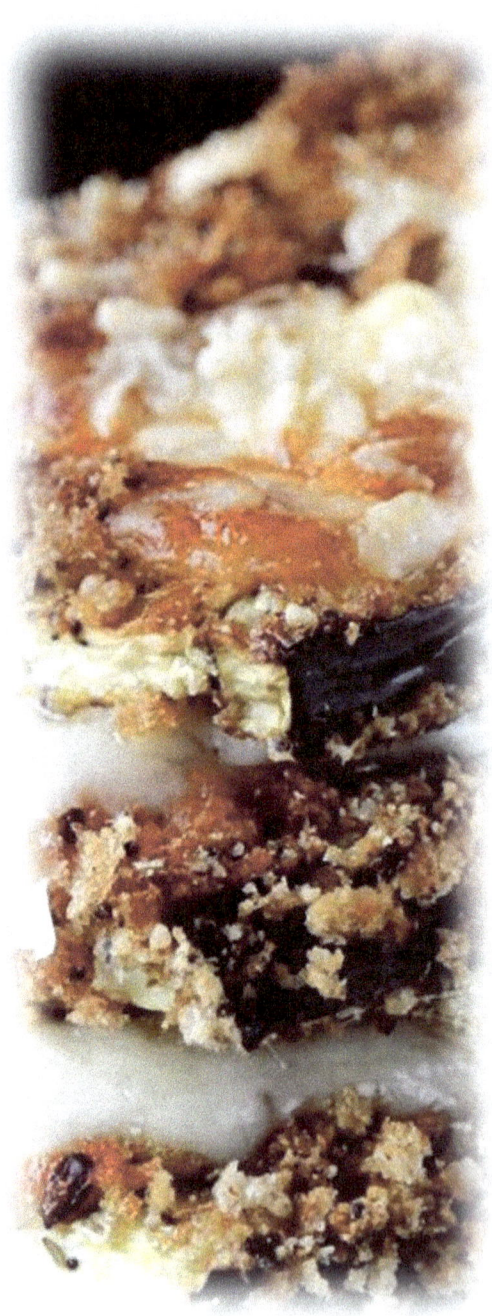

Cooking Techniques to Enhance Flavor Without Sacrificing Nutrition

- Grilling: Enhances flavor while reducing the need for added fats.
- Example: Grilled Salmon with Asparagus (high protein, omega-3 fatty acids).
- Baking: Retains nutrients and reduces the need for excess oil.
- Example: Baked Chicken Breast with Quinoa and Spinach (balanced protein and fiber).
- Stir-frying: Quick cooking method that preserves the nutritional content of vegetables.
- Example: Beef and Broccoli Stir-Fry (high protein, antioxidants).
- Steaming: Retains the nutritional value of vegetables without added fats.
- Example: Steamed Vegetables with Tofu (high in plant-based protein and fiber).
- Sautéing: Uses minimal oil and allows for quick, nutritious meals.
- Example: Sautéed Spinach with Garlic (rich in iron and vitamins).

Avoided Hearty Mains

Fried Chicken with Mashed Potatoes
- **Why to Avoid:** High in unhealthy fats and refined carbs, leading to blood sugar spikes and weight gain.

Spaghetti Carbonara
- **Why to Avoid:** High in refined carbs and saturated fats, causing rapid blood sugar spikes and increased cholesterol levels.

Beef Stroganoff
- **Why to Avoid:** High in unhealthy fats and refined carbs, contributing to poor blood sugar control and weight gain.

Cheeseburger and Fries
- **Why to Avoid:** High in refined carbs, unhealthy fats, and calories, leading to blood sugar spikes and weight gain.

Chicken Alfredo Pasta
- **Why to Avoid:** High in refined carbs and saturated fats, causing rapid blood sugar spikes and increased calorie intake.

SNACKS, SIDES, AND SWEETS

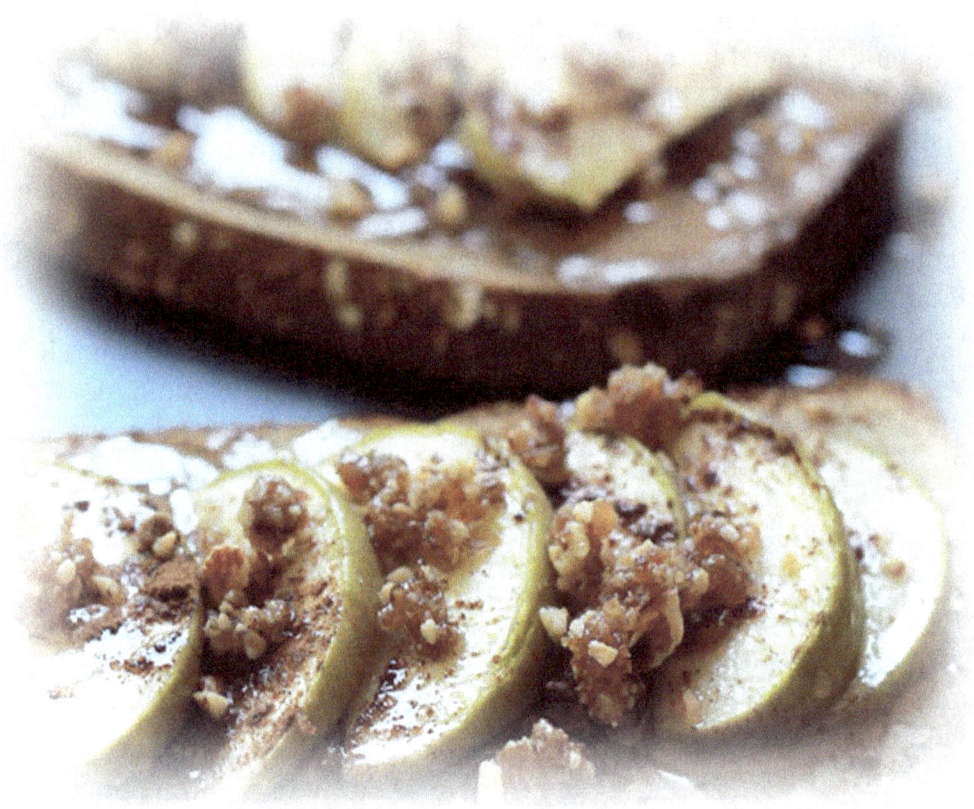

Managing prediabetes doesn't mean giving up snacks, side dishes, or sweets. Instead, it's about making intelligent choices that support stable blood sugar levels and overall health. This chapter provides a variety of nutritious and delicious recipes for snacks, sides, and sweets that fit nicely into a balanced diet. Let get started

Wholesome Snack Ideas to Keep Blood Sugar Stable Between Meals

Hummus with Veggie Sticks

- **Carb Count:** 15g
- **Nutritional Value Count and Balance:** 120 calories, 5g protein, 6g fat, 15g carbs
- **Serving Size:** 1/2 cup hummus with assorted veggies
- **Prep Time:** 10 minutes

Ingredients:
- 1/2 cup hummus
- 1 cup of mixed vegetable sticks (bell peppers, carrots, and celery)

Directions:
- Arrange veggie sticks and serve with hummus.

Health Benefit: High in fiber and plant-based protein, supporting digestive health and satiety.

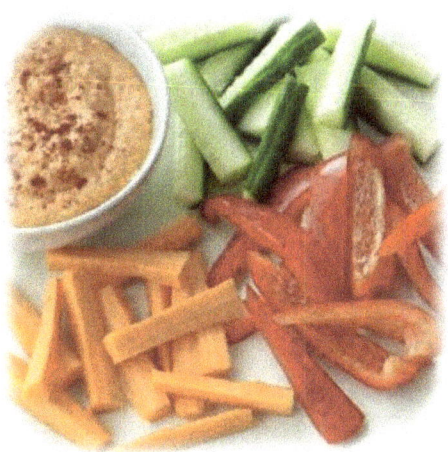

Cottage Cheese with Pineapple

- **Carb Count:** 15g
- **Nutritional Value Count and Balance:** 160 calories, 12g protein, 5g fat, 15g carbs
- **Serving Size:** 1 cup
- **Prep Time:** 5 minutes

Ingredients:
- 1 cup cottage cheese
- 1/2 cup pineapple chunks

Directions:
- Mix cottage cheese with pineapple chunks.

Health Benefit: High in protein and vitamin C, supporting muscle health and immune function.

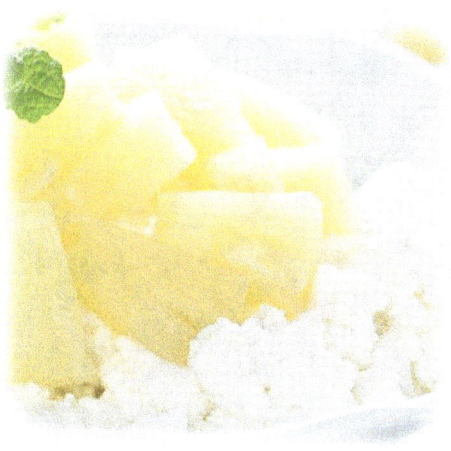

Greek Yogurt with Berries

- **Carb Count:** 12g
- **Nutritional Value Count and Balance:** 150 calories, 10g protein, 3g fat, 12g carbs
- **Serving Size:** 1 cup
- **Prep Time:** 5 minutes

Ingredients:
- 1 cup Greek yogurt (unsweetened)
- 1/2 cup mixed berries

Directions:
- Combine Greek yogurt with mixed berries in a bowl.

Health Benefit: High in protein and antioxidants, supporting gut health and stable blood sugar levels.

Almonds and Apple Slices

- **Carb Count:** 20g
- **Nutritional Value Count and Balance**: 200 calories, 5g protein, 15g fat, 20g carbs
- **Serving Size:** 1 apple with 1/4 cup almonds
- **Prep Time:** 5 minutes

Ingredients:
- 1 apple, sliced
- 1/4 cup almonds

Directions:
- Slice the apple and serve with almonds.

Health Benefit: Provides fiber and healthy fats, helping to maintain stable blood sugar levels.

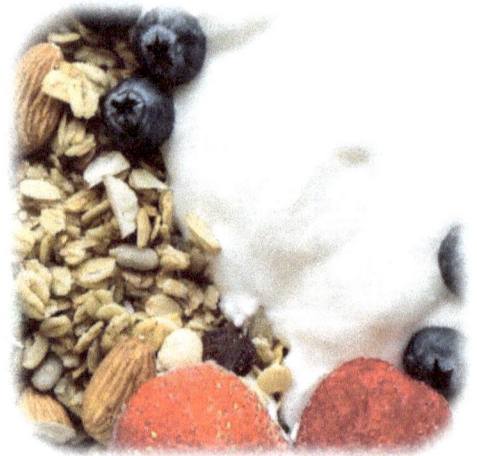
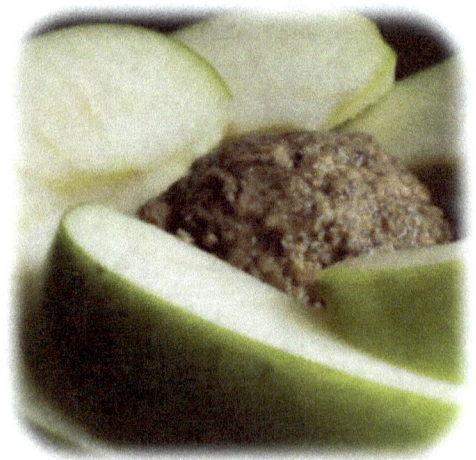

Trail Mix

- **Carb Count:** 18g
- **Nutritional Value Count and Balance:** 200 calories, 6g protein, 12g fat, 18g carbs
- **Serving Size:** 1/4 cup
- **Prep Time:** 5 minutes

Ingredients:
- 2 tbsp almonds
- 2 tbsp walnuts
- 2 tbsp dried cranberries (unsweetened)

Directions:
- Mix all ingredients in a bowl.

Health Benefit: Provides a mix of healthy fats, protein, and fiber, supporting energy and blood sugar control.

Avoided Snacks

Chips and Dip
- **Why to Avoid:** High in unhealthy fats and refined carbs, leading to blood sugar spikes and weight gain.

Candy Bars
- **Why to Avoid:** High in sugar and empty calories, causing rapid blood sugar spikes.

Pretzels
- **Why to Avoid:** High in refined carbs and low in nutrients, leading to blood sugar fluctuations.

Sugary Granola Bars
- Why to Avoid: High in sugar and low in protein, causing rapid blood sugar spikes.

Flavored Yogurts
- Why to Avoid: High in added sugars, leading to blood sugar spikes and weight gain.

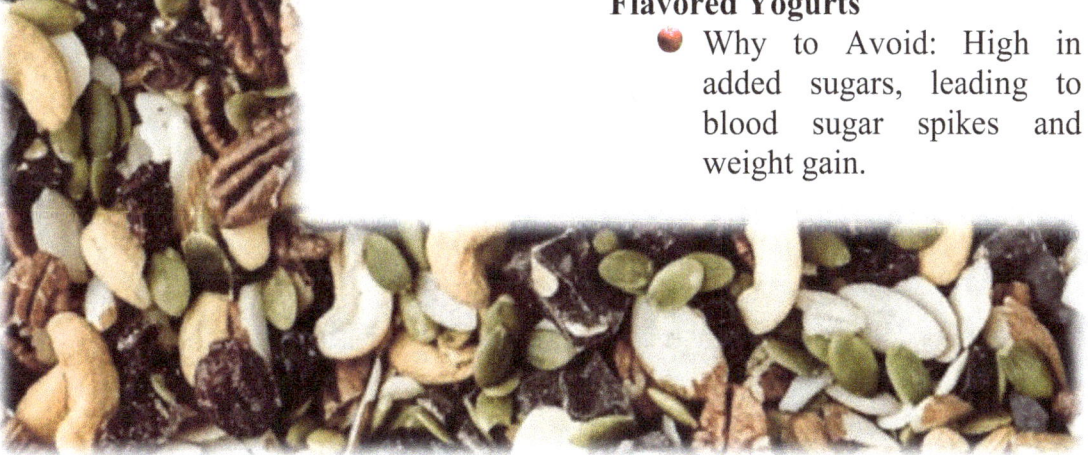

Flavorful Side Dish Recipes to Complement Any Meal

Roasted Brussels Sprouts

- **Carb Count:** 15g
- **Nutritional Value Count and Balance:** 150 calories, 4g protein, 8g fat, 15g carbs
- **Serving Size:** 1 cup
- **Prep Time:** 25 minutes

Ingredients:
- 2 cups Brussels sprouts, halved
- 2 tbsp olive oil
- Salt and pepper to taste

Directions:
- Preheat oven to 400°F.
- Toss Brussels sprouts with olive oil, salt, and pepper.
- Roast for 20-25 minutes until crispy.

Health Benefit: Rich in fiber and antioxidants, supporting digestive health and reducing inflammation.

Sweet Potato Fries

- **Carb Count:** 30g
- **Nutritional Value Count and Balance:** 180 calories, 2g protein, 5g fat, 30g carbs
- **Serving Size:** 1 cup
- **Prep Time:** 30 minutes

Ingredients:
- 2 sweet potatoes cut into fries
- 2 tbsp olive oil
- Salt and paprika to taste

Directions:
- Preheat oven to 425°F.
- Add salt, paprika, and olive oil to sweet potatoes and toss.
- Bake for 25-30 minutes until crispy.

Health Benefit: High in fiber and beta-carotene, supporting vision and blood sugar control.

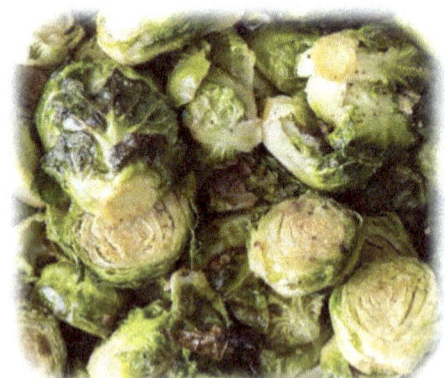

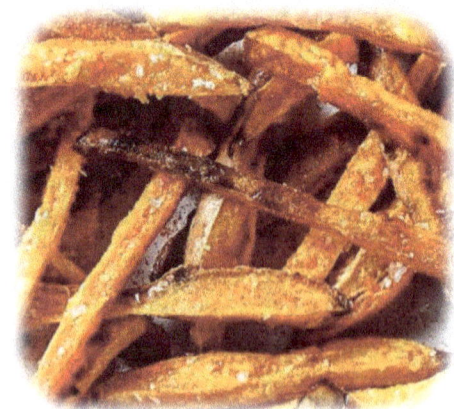

Garlic Green Beans

- **Carb Count:** 10g
- **Nutritional Value Count and Balance:** 80 calories, 2g protein, 4g fat, 10g carbs
- **Serving Size:** 1 cup
- **Prep Time:** 15 minutes

Ingredients:
- 2 cups green beans
- 2 cloves garlic, minced
- 1 tbsp olive oil

Directions:
- Heat olive oil in a pan over medium heat.
- Add garlic and green beans, and sauté until tender.

Health Benefit: High in vitamins A and C, supporting immune function and overall health.

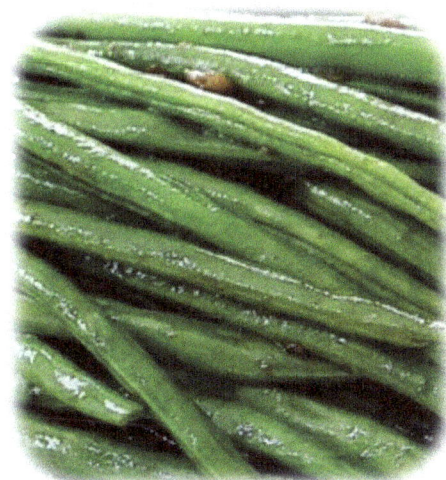

Cauliflower Rice

- **Carb Count: 5g**
- **Nutritional Value Count and Balance:** 50 calories, 2g protein, 2g fat, 5g carbs
- **Serving Size:** 1 cup
- **Prep Time:** 10 minutes

Ingredients:
- 1 head cauliflower, grated
- 1 tbsp olive oil
- Salt and pepper to taste

Directions:
- Over medium heat, warm up some olive oil in a pan. Add grated cauliflower, salt, and pepper.
- Sauté for 5-7 minutes until tender.

Health Benefit: Low in carbs and high in fiber, supporting weight management and blood sugar stability.

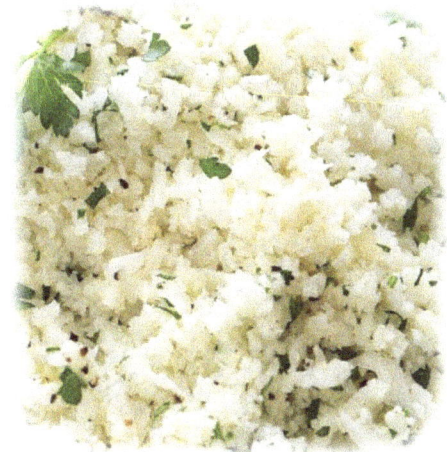

Quinoa Salad with Avocado

- **Carb Count:** 25g
- **Nutritional Value Count and Balance:** 220 calories, 8g protein, 10g fat, 25g carbs
- **Serving Size:** 1 cup
- **Prep Time:** 20 minutes

Ingredients:
- 1 cup cooked quinoa
- 1/2 avocado, diced
- 1/4 cup cherry tomatoes, halved
- 1 tbsp olive oil
- 1 tbsp lemon juice

Directions:
- In a bowl, combine all the ingredients and healthy mix.

Health Benefit: High in healthy fats and fiber, supporting heart health and digestion.

Avoided Sides

Mashed Potatoes with Gravy
- **Why to Avoid:** High in refined carbs and unhealthy fats, causing rapid blood sugar spikes.

Fried Onion Rings
- Why to Avoid: High in unhealthy fats and refined carbs, leading to blood sugar spikes and weight gain.

Creamed Spinach
- **Why to Avoid:** High in unhealthy fats and calories, contributing to poor blood sugar control.

Buttered Corn
- **Why to Avoid:** High in refined carbs and added fats, causing rapid blood sugar spikes.

Macaroni and Cheese
- **Why to Avoid:** High in refined carbs and unhealthy fats, leading to blood sugar spikes and weight gain.

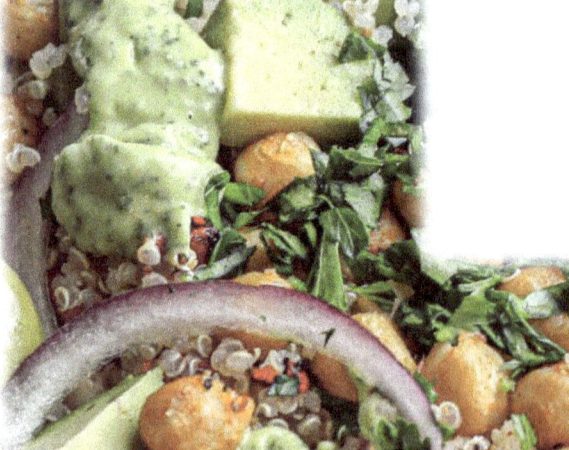

Indulgent Dessert Options for Occasional Treats

Dark Chocolate Avocado Mousse

- **Carb Count:** 15g
- **Nutritional Value Count and Balance:** 200 calories, 3g protein, 15g fat, 15g carbs
- **Serving Size:** 1/2 cup
- **Prep Time:** 10 minutes

Ingredients:
- 1 ripe avocado
- 2 tbsp cocoa powder
- 2 tbsp honey or maple syrup

Directions:
- Blend all ingredients until smooth.
- Chill before serving.

Health Benefit: Rich in healthy fats and antioxidants, supporting heart health and satiety.

Chia Seed Pudding

- **Carb Count:** 20g
- **Nutritional Value Count and Balance:** 150 calories, 5g protein, 8g fat, 20g carbs
- **Serving Size:** 1/2 cup
- **Prep Time:** 10 minutes (+ overnight chilling)

Ingredients:
- 1/4 cup chia seeds
- 1 cup almond milk
- 1 tbsp honey or maple syrup

Directions:
- Mix all ingredients in a bowl.
- Chill overnight until thickened.

Health Benefit: High in fiber and omega-3 fatty acids, supporting digestive health and reducing inflammation.

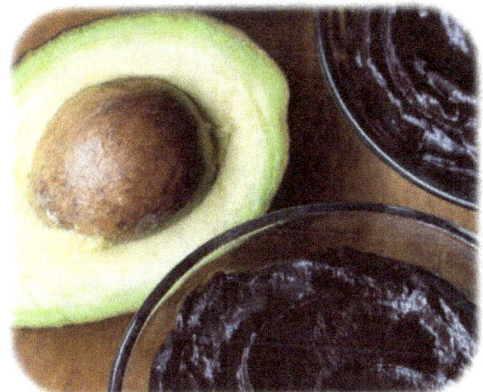
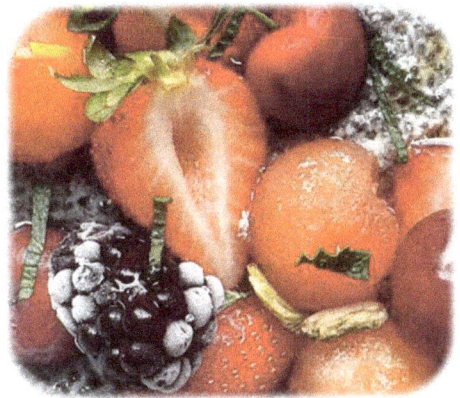

Greek Yogurt with Honey and Nuts

- **Carb Count:** 15g
- **Nutritional Value Count and Balance:** 200 calories, 10g protein, 10g fat, 15g carbs
- **Serving Size:** 1 cup
- **Prep Time:** 5 minutes

Ingredients:
- 1 cup Greek yogurt
- 1 tbsp honey
- 2 tbsp mixed nuts

Directions:
- Combine all ingredients in a bowl.

Health Benefit: High protein and healthy fats, supporting muscle health and satiety.

Baked Apple with Cinnamon

- **Carb Count:** 20g
- **Nutritional Value Count and Balance:** 120 calories, 1g protein, 2g fat, 20g carbs
- **Serving Size: 1 apple**
- **Prep Time:** 30 minutes

Ingredients:
- 1 apple, cored
- 1 tbsp honey
- 1 tsp cinnamon

Directions:
- Preheat oven to 350°F.
- Fill apple with honey and cinnamon.
- Bake for 25-30 minutes until tender.

Health Benefit: High in fiber and antioxidants, supporting digestion and reducing inflammation.

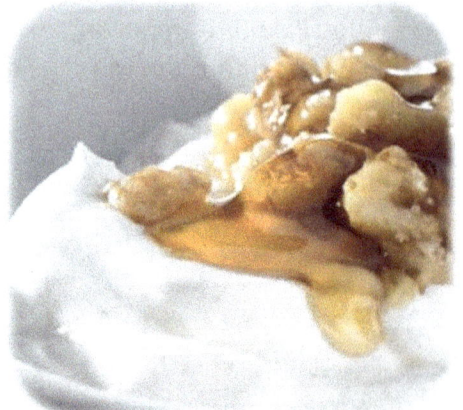
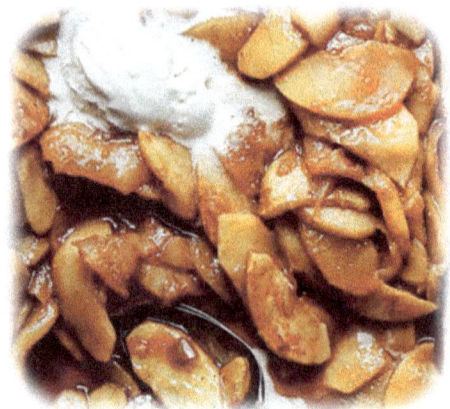

Coconut Macaroons

- **Carb Count:** 10g
- **Nutritional Value Count and Balance:** 100 calories, 1g protein, 7g fat, 10g carbs
- **Serving Size:** 2 macaroons
- **Prep Time:** 20 minutes

Ingredients:
- 1 cup shredded coconut
- 1/4 cup honey
- 1 egg white

Directions:
- Preheat oven to 325°F.
- Mix all ingredients in a bowl.
- Scoop onto a baking sheet and bake for 15-20 minutes.

Health Benefit: Low in carbs and high in healthy fats, supporting satiety and stable blood sugar levels.

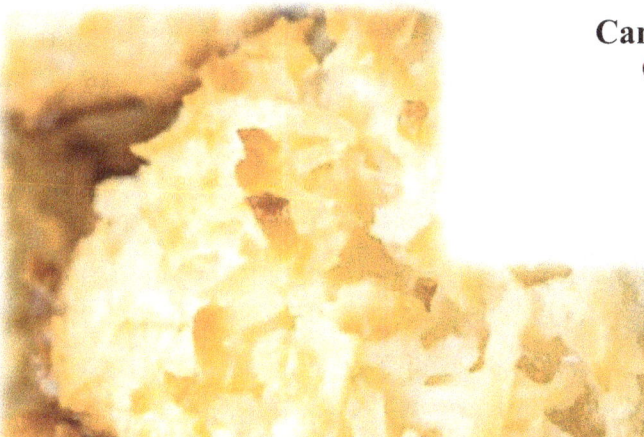

Avoided Sweets

Ice Cream
- **Why to Avoid:** High in sugar and unhealthy fats, causing rapid blood sugar spikes.

Cookies
- **Why to Avoid:** High in sugar and refined carbs, leading to blood sugar fluctuations.

Cake
- **Why to Avoid:** High in sugar and refined carbs, causing rapid blood sugar spikes.

Doughnuts
- **Why to Avoid**: High in sugar, unhealthy fats, and refined carbs, leading to blood sugar spikes and weight gain.

Candy
- **Why to Avoid:** High in sugar and empty calories, causing rapid blood sugar spikes.

CONCLUSION

Now that we have completed our journey through the management of prediabetes, let's pause to consider the essential ideas and tactics we have discussed and discover the will to maintain these long-term healthy behaviors.

Recap of Key Concepts and Strategies for Prediabetes Reversal: Throughout this guide, we've dug into various aspects of prediabetes, from understanding its definition and implications to exploring nutrition, exercise, and lifestyle interventions. We've learned the importance of balanced meals, regular physical activity, stress management, quality sleep, and mindfulness practices in managing blood sugar levels and promoting overall health. By implementing these strategies, individuals with prediabetes can take proactive steps toward reversing the condition and reducing their risk of developing type 2 diabetes and other related complications.

Encouragement and Motivation for Sustaining Healthy Habits Long-Term: Reversing prediabetes demands perseverance and commitment. Nevertheless, it's critical to remember that development isn't necessarily linear. Despite obstacles, every step you take in the right direction will help you reach your objectives. Acknowledging and appreciating your accomplishments, no matter how tiny, and cultivating self-compassion in trying times is critical.

Recall that you are traveling with others. Seek assistance from friends, family, and medical experts who can offer support, accountability, and direction. Additionally, pursue interests and hobbies that make you happy and fulfilled. Long-term maintenance of healthy behaviors depends on leading a balanced and pleasurable lifestyle.

Remaining consistent and persistent is crucial as you proceed with your prediabetes reversal quest. You may enhance your well-being and lower your risk of chronic disease by adopting durable and gradual adjustments to your food, exercise regimen, and way of life. Remain focused and motivated, and keep in mind that each healthy decision you make moves you one step closer to reaching your objectives.

www.ingramcontent.com/pod-product-compliance
Lightning Source LLC
Chambersburg PA
CBHW062315220526
45479CB00004B/1182